· 四川大学精品立项教材 ·

PRE-CLINIC TRAINING GUIDE ON PEDIATRIC DENTISTRY

儿童口腔医学临床前实验指导

主　编　邹　静
副主编　周　媛
编　者（按姓氏拼音排序）
黄睿洁　刘人恺　马　佳　蒙明梅
彭怡然　舒　睿　王　了　王　艳
杨　燃　周陈晨　邹　静　张　琼
周　昕　周　媛

四川大學出版社
Sichuan University Press

项目策划：龚娇梅
责任编辑：龚娇梅
责任校对：张　澄
封面设计：墨创文化
责任印制：王　炜

图书在版编目（CIP）数据

儿童口腔医学临床前实验指导 ：英文 / 邹静主编
. — 成都 ：四川大学出版社，2020.6
ISBN 978-7-5690-3772-2

Ⅰ．①儿… Ⅱ．①邹… Ⅲ．①小儿疾病－口腔疾病－诊疗－英文 Ⅳ．①R788

中国版本图书馆 CIP 数据核字（2020）第 108507 号

书名　儿童口腔医学临床前实验指导
Ertong Kouqiang Yixue Linchuang qian Shiyan Zhidao

主　　编	邹　静
出　　版	四川大学出版社
地　　址	成都市一环路南一段 24 号（610065）
发　　行	四川大学出版社
书　　号	ISBN 978-7-5690-3772-2
印前制作	四川胜翔数码印务设计有限公司
印　　刷	成都市新都华兴印务有限公司
成品尺寸	185mm×260mm
印　　张	7
字　　数	220 千字
版　　次	2020 年 12 月第 1 版
印　　次	2020 年 12 月第 1 次印刷
定　　价	32.00 元

◆ 读者邮购本书，请与本社发行科联系。
电话：(028)85408408/(028)85401670/
(028)86408023　邮政编码：610065
◆ 本社图书如有印装质量问题，请寄回出版社调换。
◆ 网址：http://press.scu.edu.cn

四川大学出版社
微信公众号

Introduction

Pediatric dentistry is an age-defined specialty that provides both primary and comprehensive preventive and therapeutic oral health care for infants and children through adolescence, including those with special health needs.

By being an age-specific specialty, pediatric dentistry encompasses disciplines such as behavior guidance, supervision of orofacial growth and development, caries risk assessment and prevention, sedation, space maintenance for early loss of primary molars, early intervention of malocclusion, orofacial muscle training for oral habits of children, as well as other traditional fields of dentistry. These skills are applied to the oral health care of children throughout their ever-changing stages of development and treating conditions and diseases unique to growing individuals. To become a pediatric dental specialist, a dentist must complete this comprehensive pre-clinic training program designed to provide specialized knowledge and skills before facing the children and adolescence in pediatric dental clinics.

This pre-clinic training guide on pediatric dentistry includes six major sections: i. morphology of the primary and immature permanent tooth, ii. radiographic diagnostics in pediatric dentistry, iii. caries risk assessment and oral health instruction, iv. behavior guidance, v. techniques in restoration for primary teeth, vi. occlusive guidance in pediatric dentistry.

CONTENTS

CHAPTER 1

MORPHOLOGY AND RADIOGRAPHIC CHARACTERISTICS OF THE PRIMARY AND IMMATURE PERMANENT TEETH

Introduction to the morphology of the primary and immature permanent teeth

Primary teeth, also known as deciduous teeth, milk teeth, baby teeth and temporary teeth, are the first set of teeth in the growth development of humans. They develop during the embryonic stage of development and erupt—that is, they become visible in the mouth—during infancy. They are usually lost and replaced by permanent teeth, but in the absence of permanent replacements, they can remain functional for many years.

Permanent teeth or adult teeth are the second set of teeth of humans. In humans and old-world simians, there are 32 permanent teeth, consisting of six maxillary and six mandibular molars, four maxillary and four mandibular premolars, two maxillary and two mandibular canines, four maxillary and four mandibular incisors. The first permanent tooth usually appears in the mouth at around six years of age, and the mouth will then be in a transition time with both primary teeth and permanent teeth during the mixed dentition period until the last primary tooth is lost or shed. The first of the permanent teeth to erupt are the permanent first molars, right behind the last primary second molars of the primary dentition. These first permanent molars are important for the correct development of the permanent dentition. Up to the age of thirteen years, 28 of the 32 permanent teeth will appear. The full permanent dentition is completed much later during the permanent dentition period. The four last permanent teeth, the third molars, usually appear between the ages of 17 and 38; they are considered wisdom teeth.

In 1895 Wilhelm Conrad Rontgen discovered X-rays, a form of high-energy electromagnetic radiation. This technique has been applied in dentistry since 1896, and it provides a very significant advantage to the dental and maxillofacial diagnosis. Two-dimensional intraoral radiography and extraoral radiography are the two traditional techniques. Besides, as the development of new techniques, Cone Beam Computed Tomography (CBCT) has been widely used in recent years. However, due to the relatively large dose of radiation, discontinuous image capture and high expense, CBCT is not the first choice of radiographic examination in

Pediatric Dentistry. It is mainly used in obtaining the spatial information of an impacted tooth for instance.

Tooth notation systems

Palmer notation for permanent teeth (Figure 1 -1).

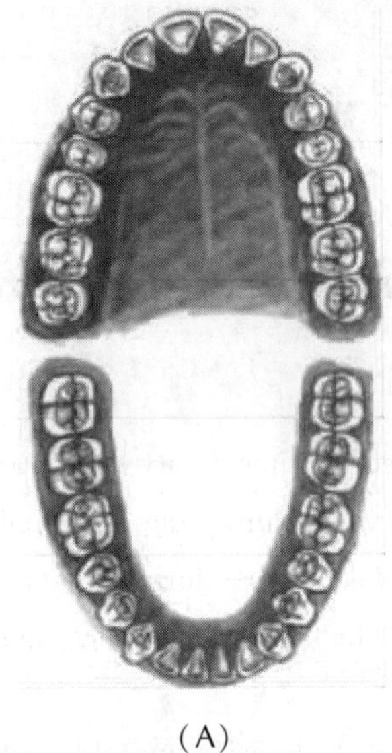

(A)

87654321	12345678
87654321	12345678

(B)

Figure 1 -1

Palmer notation for primary teeth (Figure 1 -2).

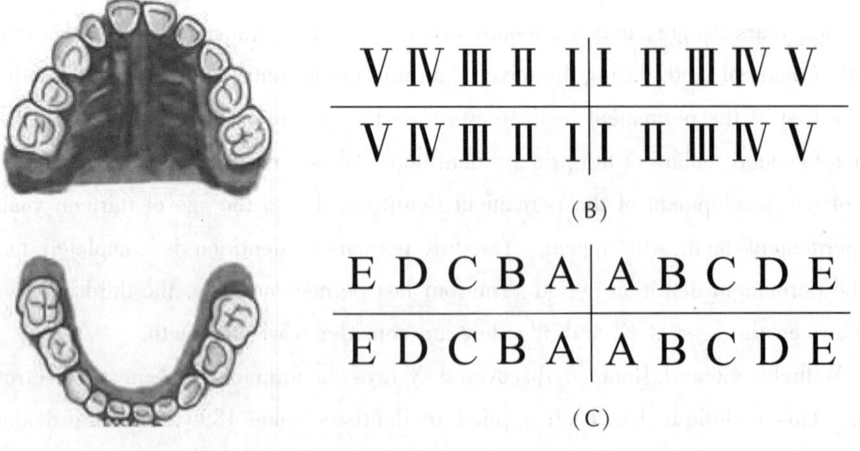

(A)

Figure 1 -2

Federation Dentaire International (FDI) notation for permanent teeth (Figure 1-3).

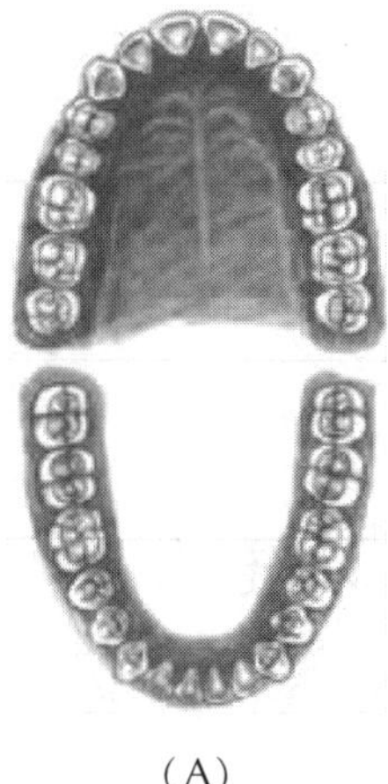

(A)

18	17	16	15	14	13	12	11	21	22	23	24	25	26	27	28
48	47	46	45	44	43	42	41	31	32	33	34	35	36	37	38

(B)

Figure 1-3

Federation Dentaire International (FDI) notation for primary teeth (Figure 1-4).

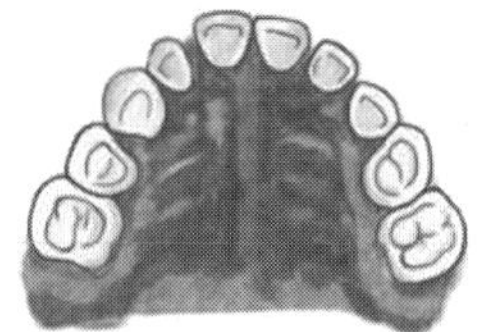

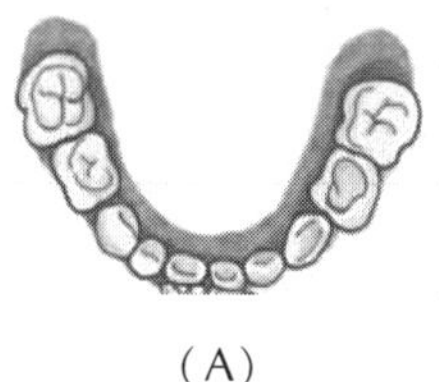

(A)

55	54	53	52	51	61	62	63	64	65
85	84	83	82	81	71	72	73	74	75

(B)

Figure 1-4

Universal notation system for the permanent teeth (Figure 1-5).

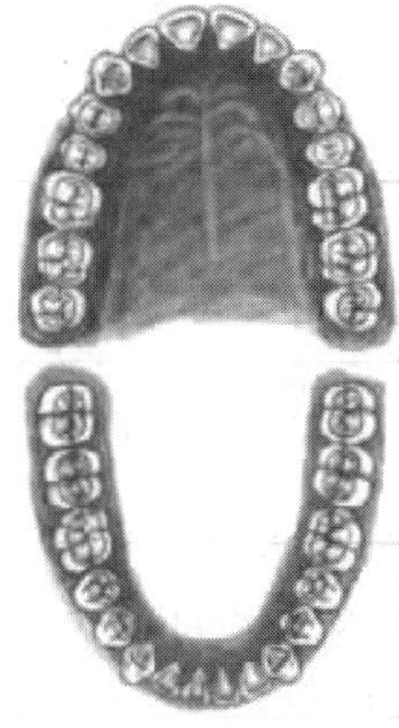

(A)

1	2	3	4	5	6	7	8	9	10	11	12	13	14	15	16
32	31	30	29	28	27	26	25	24	23	22	21	20	19	18	17

(B)

Figure 1-5

Universal notation system for primary teeth (Figure 1 -6).

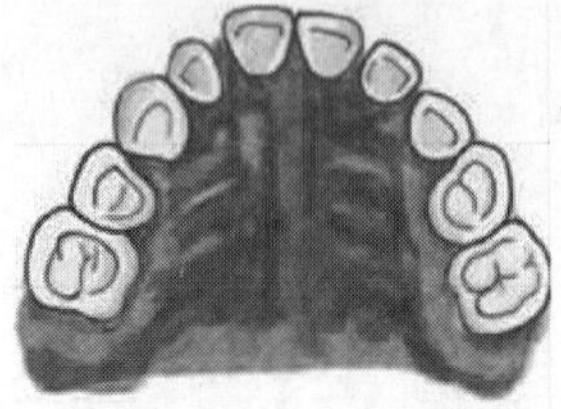

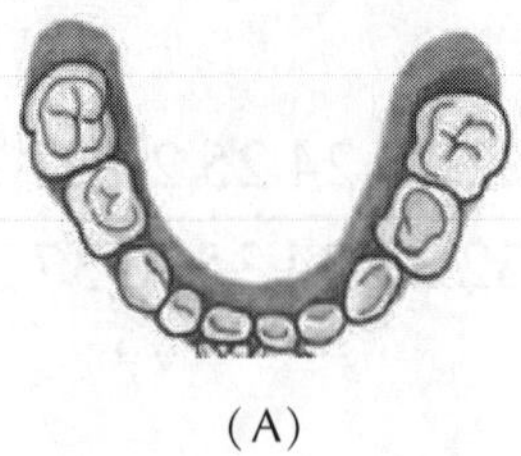

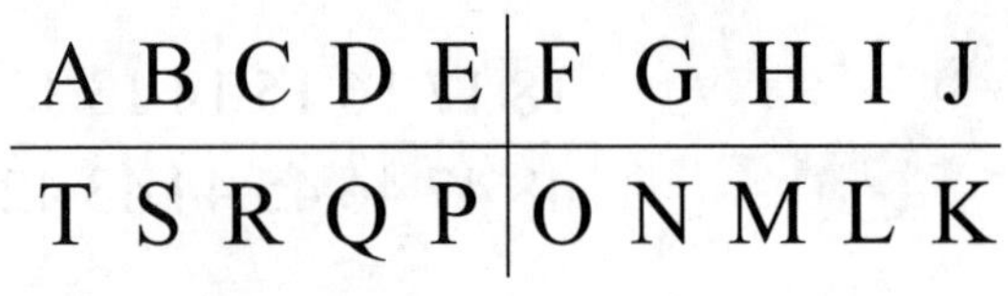

(A) (B)

Figure 1 -6

Characteristics of primary teeth

Characteristics of primary teeth including:

- Smaller in size than the analogous permanent teeth.
- Whiter in color than permanent teeth.
- Less mineralized.
- Enamel and dentin are approximately one half the thickness of their analogous permanent teeth.
- Shorter crowns with respect to roots. In other words, they have greater root-to-crown length ratio.
- Crowns have a marked constriction at the CEJ.
- Crowns seem to bulge rather than taper near the cervical lines.
- Crowns appear bulbous, often having labial or buccal cingula.
- Significantly shallower coronal anatomy compared to their analogous permanent teeth.

In general, primary teeth have rounded cusps and they lack secondary featuresr.

- More consistent shapes than their analogous permanent teeth (i. e. fewer anomalies).
- Pulp cavities are proportionally larger than their analogous permanent teeth.

It is important to differentiate primary teeth and permanent teeth by comparing the tooth crown size, relative crown size in the arch, color, mineralization, enamel thickness, dentin thickness, root-to-crown ration, cervical constriction, coronal anatomy, pulp chamber, pulp horn, root trunk, root furcation, root canals and accessory canals (Table 1 -1, Figure 1 -7).

Table 1 – 1 Tooth morphology and radiographic characters comparison between primary teeth and permanent teeth.

	Primary teeth	Permanent teeth
Crown size	Smaller	Bigger
Relative crown size in the arch	First molar < second molar	First molar > second molar
Color	Whitish	Yellowish
Mineralization	Less	More
Enamel thickness	Thinner	Thicker
Dentin thickness	Thinner	Thicker
Root-to-crown ration	Smaller	Greater
Cervical constriction	Obviously marked	Not well-marked
Coronal anatomy	Shallow	Deep
Pulp chamber	Relatively large	Relatively small
Pulp horn	Higher	Lower
Root trunk	Smaller	Larger
Root furcation	Obtuse angle	Acute angle
Root canals	Short and wide	Long and narrow
Accessory canals	Present	May be absent

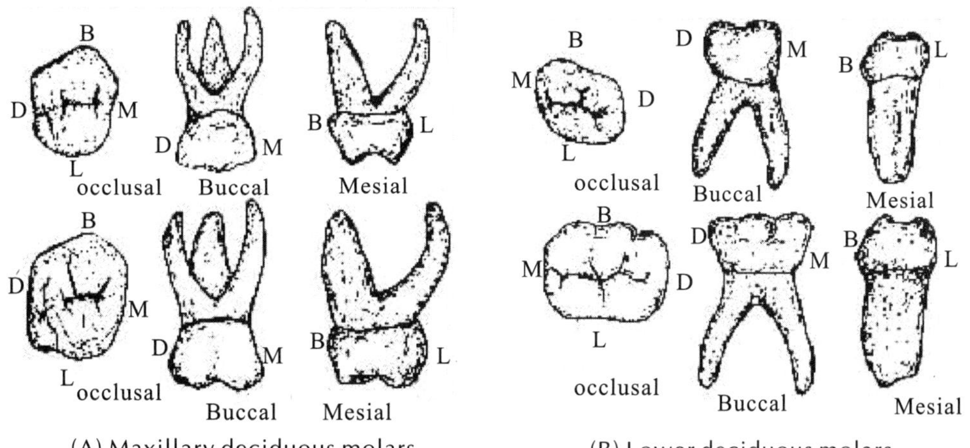

Figure 1 –7 Morphology comparison between the primary first molar and the permanent first molar.

Radiographic techniques

Periapical radiography

It should show the crown of the tooth and at least 3mm beyond the apex of the tooth. Both the paralleling technique and bisecting angle technique can be used, but the paralleling technique is preferred because of its accuracy.

Bitewing radiography

It is intended to assess interproximal caries and interproximal bone height. Paralleling technique is used to obtain bitewing films.

Panoramic radiography

The panoramic image is obtained through tomography. This means that only the structures located in the focal trough are captured in focus. The images are like bitewing images but magnified.

Cone beam computed tomography (CBCT)

It is ideal for imaging hard tissues and provides the three-dimensional information of the craniofacial structures.

Nolla's stage of tooth calcification

Nolla's stage of tooth calcification is also known as Nolla's stage of tooth development. Nolla has divided the stages of tooth development into ten stages (Figure 1 -8):

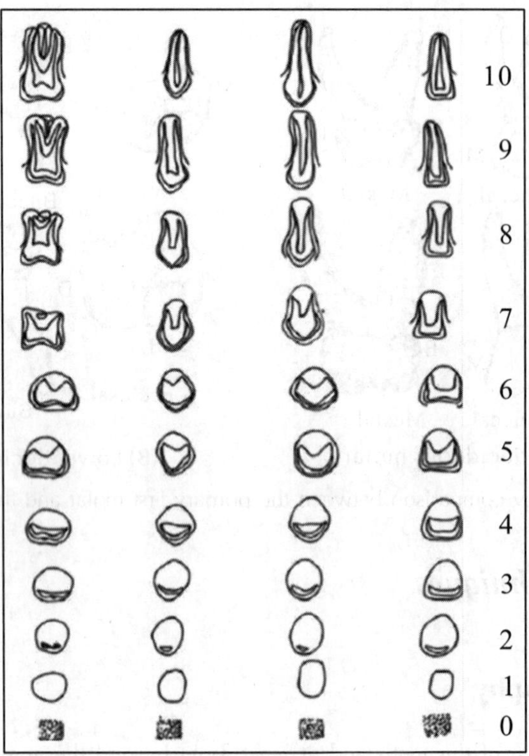

Figure 1 -8 Nolla's stage of tooth calcification.

0—Absence of crypt
1—Presence of crypt
2—Initial calcification
3—1/3 of crown completed
4—2/3 of crown completed
5—Crown almost completed
6—Crown completed
7—1/3 of root completed
8—2/3 of root completed
9—Root almost completed with open apex
10—Apical end of root completed

Nolla's stage of tooth calcification is widely used in assessing dental calcification and estimating tooth development.

The objective of lab practice

1. To master the morphology and radiographic differences of primary and immature permanent teeth.
2. To master the Palmer and Federation Dentaire International (FDI) tooth notation systems.
3. To be familiar with radiographic techniques.
4. To be familiar with Nolla's stages of tooth calcification.
5. To know the Universal notation systems.

Materials

1. Photos of primary teeth for demonstration.
2. Photos of permanent teeth for demonstration.
3. Photos of clinic cases.
4. Periapical films of primary and permanent teeth.
5. Bitewing films of primary and permanent teeth.
6. Panoramic films of primary and permanent teeth.
7. CBCT films of primary and permanent teeth.

Practice steps

1. Review the teeth notation systems.
2. Study the morphologic and radiographic differences between primary and immature permanent teeth.

3. Display PowerPoint slides of primary and/or immature permanent teeth are displaced on the screen to the class (Supplementary material 1). The students would have 30 minutes to recognize all the teeth.
4. The lecturer randomly picks candidate primary or immature permanent teeth from the photos and invites students to answer what teeth are they and give the reasons.
5. The lecturer judges whether the student's answer is correct or not, and gives the class feedbacks related to the teeth and the performance of the student.
6. Quiz of 10 photos of teeth is displayed to the class, and the students need to write down what teeth are they in 10 minutes.
7. Discuss the right answer after the collection of answer sheets.

Tips

1. Palmer notation is the system that causes the least mistake. Therefore, it is required to be mastered and highly recommended in the quiz.
2. Remember all the different characters listed in Table 1 - 1 before you start the quiz.
3. Compare the sizes of lateral incisor and canine, if the size of lateral incisor is larger than canine, then, the lateral incisor is a permanent tooth while the canine is a primary tooth.
4. If there are two rows of teeth, this is either primary dentition or mixed dentition.
5. In a primary dentition or mixed dentition radiography, find the canine first. Then, the molar next to canine will be the primary first molar or permanent first premolar.
6. The first permanent molar does not replace any primary tooth.

Process assessment for students' practice during class

1. Randomly invite students to tell the notation of teeth in class.
2. In-class discussion performance.
3. In-class quiz.

Supplemental materials

Photos that demonstrates primary and/or immature permanent teeth for in-class tooth identification discussion.

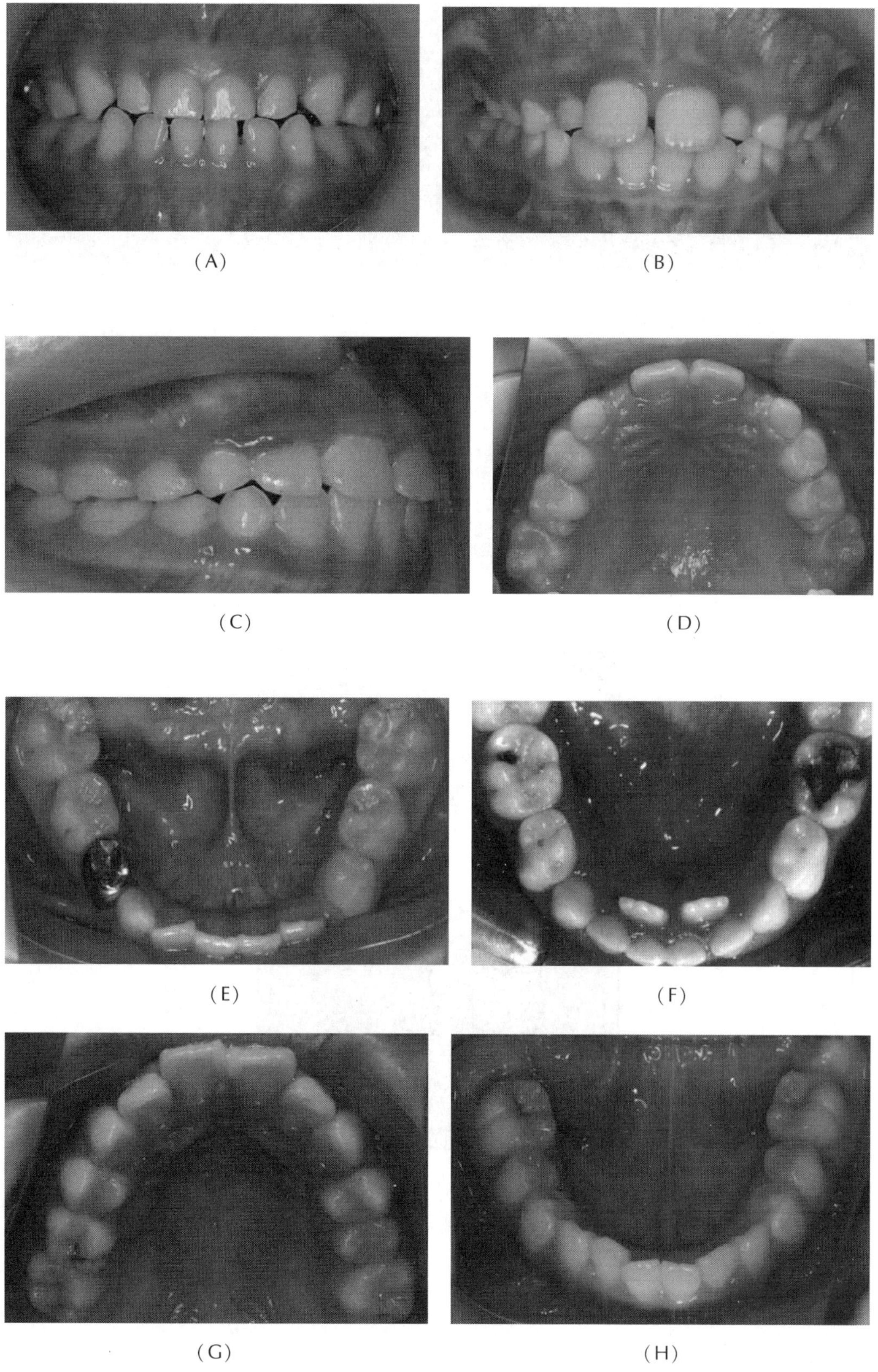

(A) (B)

(C) (D)

(E) (F)

(G) (H)

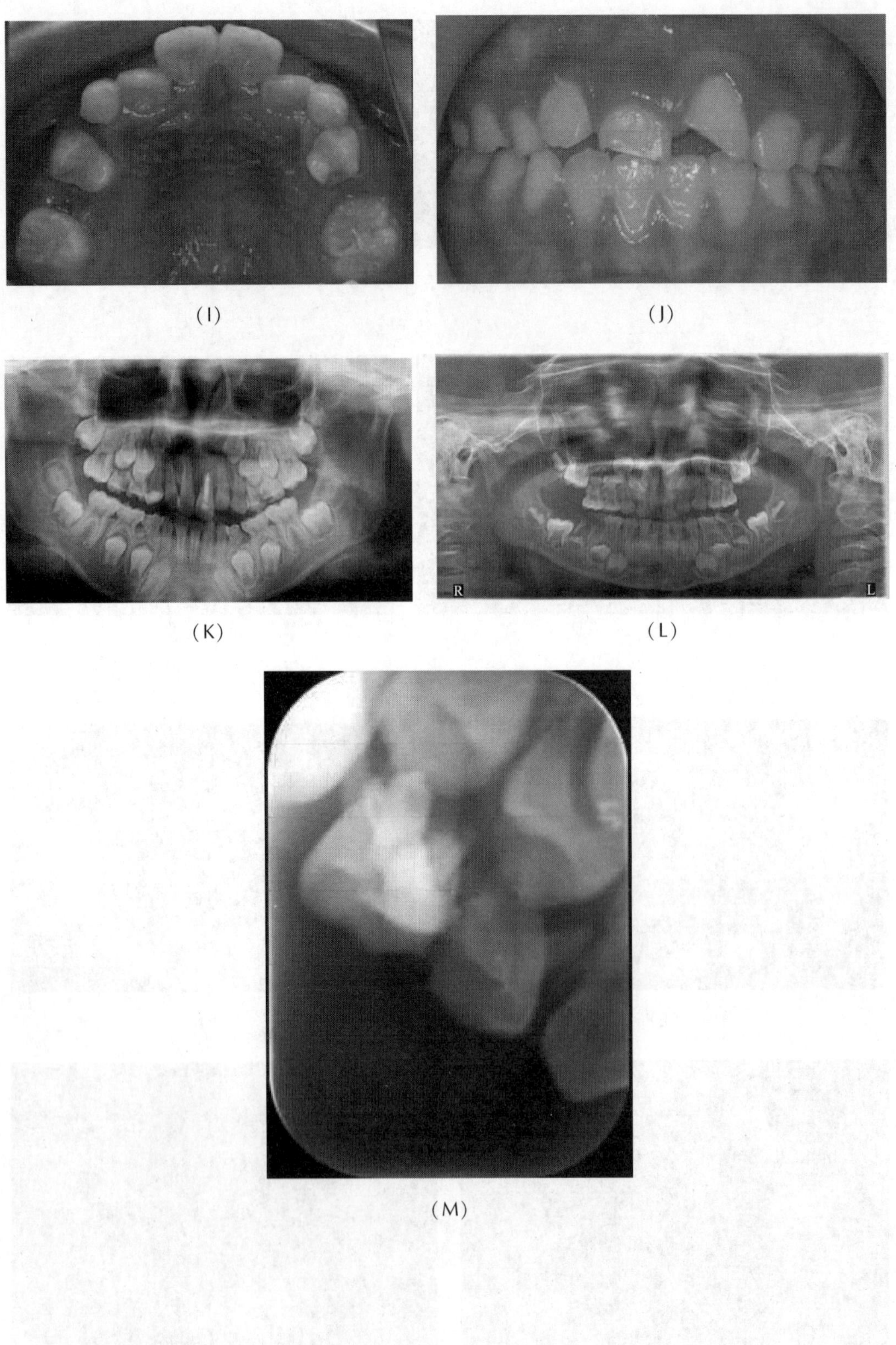

(I) (J) (K) (L) (M)

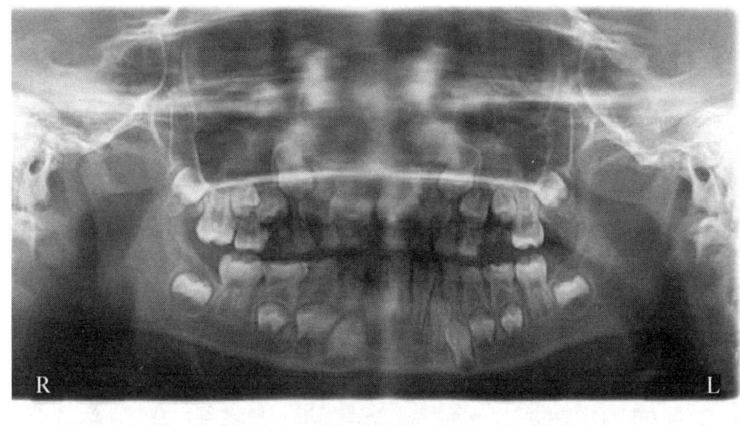

(N)

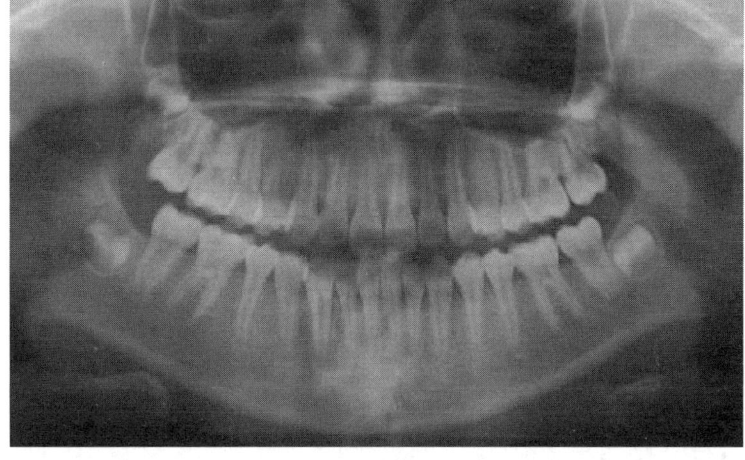

(O)

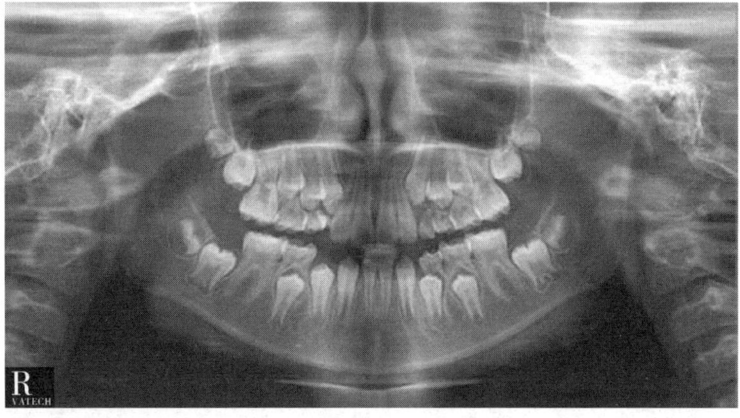

(P)

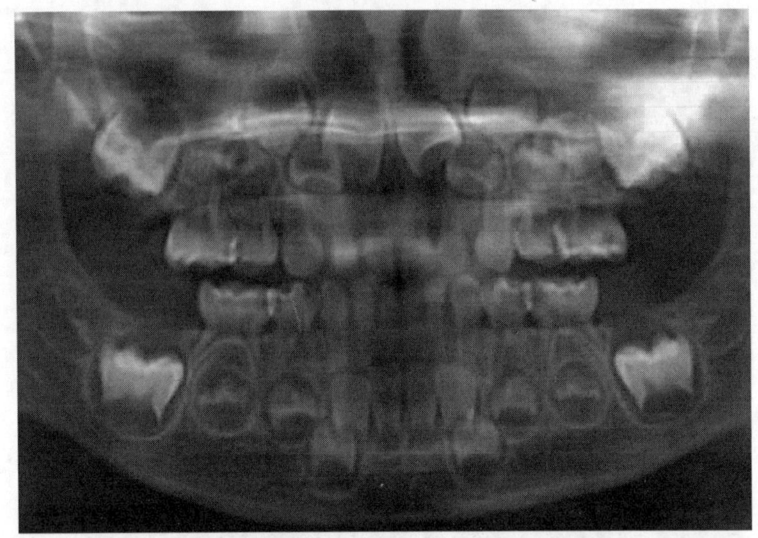

(Q)

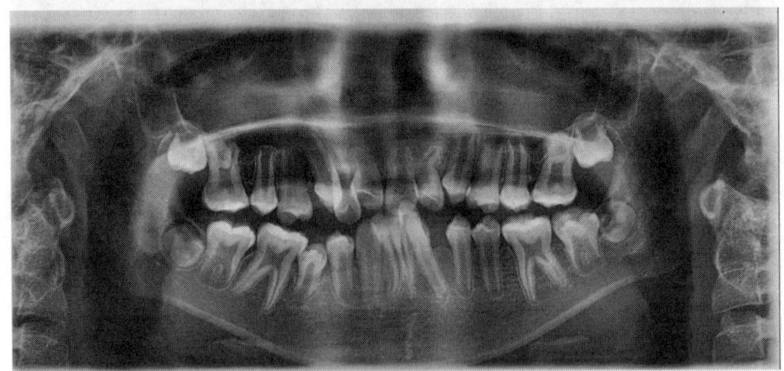

(R)

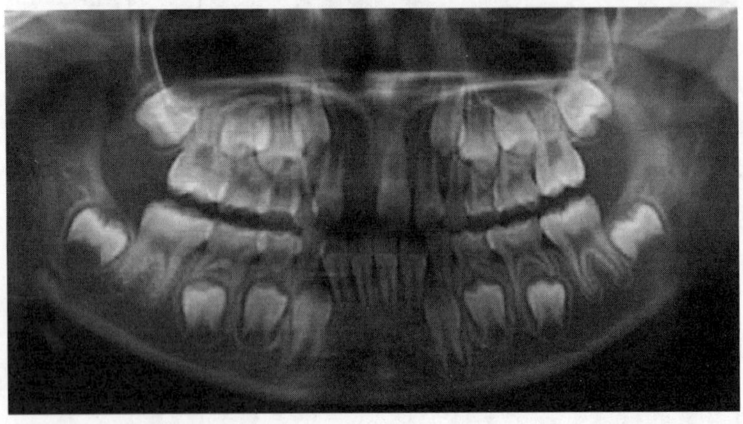

(S)

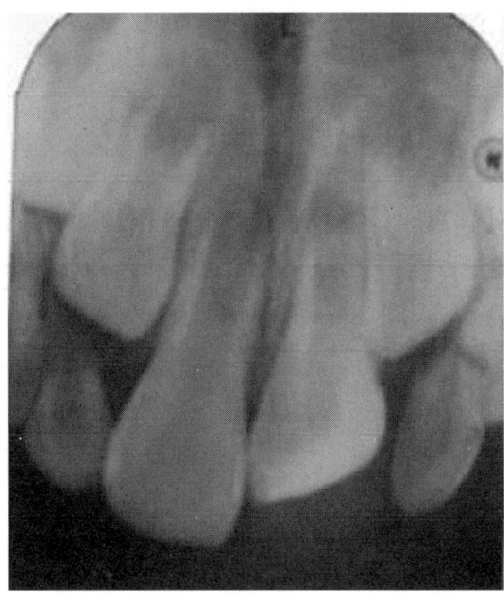

(T)

References

McDonald RE, Avery D. McDonald and Avery's dentistry for the child and adolescent [M]. 10th ed. Indianapolis: Mosby, 2016.

CHAPTER 2

CARIES RISK ASSESSMENT AND ORAL HEALTH INSTRUCTION FOR CHILDREN

Introduction to caries risk assessment tools

Caries risk assessment is the determination of the likelihood of the incidence of caries (i. e., the number of new cavitated or incipient lesions) during a certain time or the likelihood that there will be an alteration in the size or activity of lesions already existed. The assessment of caries risk in pediatric dentistry is pivotal in clinical decision making regarding the prevention and treatment protocol of dental caries for each child.

Caries-risk assessment models currently involve a combination of factors including a susceptible host, microflora, diet and fluoride exposure that interplay with a variety of cultural, social, and behavioral factors. The most used caries risk assessment tool includes Caries-Risk Assessment Tool (CAT), Caries Management by Risk Assessment (CAMBRA) and Cariogram. CAT developed by the American Academy of Pediatric Dentistry (AAPD), consists of two forms: one for children 0 - 5 years old and one for children older than 5 years (supplemental materials 1). CAMBRA was developed by the American Dental Association (ADA), including one form for patients 0 - 6 years old and one form for patients older than 6 years (supplemental materials 2). The "Cariogram" is a computer caries-risk program that records ten data points including but not limited to past caries experience, diet, oral hygiene habits, fluoride exposures and analysis of saliva (Supplemental materials 3). The program presents the results as a colored graph. The different colors are as follows: dark blue for diet, red for bacteria, yellow for circumstances, and light blue for susceptibility-related factors; green represents the chance of avoiding caries. Estimation for the chance of avoiding caries (new cavities) will be reported for dentists' reference.

The objective of lab practice

1. To recognize the significance of performing a caries risk assessment on pediatric patients.
2. To master the principles of caries management by risk assessment.

3. To be familiar with different caries risk assessment tools.
4. To know and differentiate between clinical protocols used to manage dental caries.

Materials

1. Caries assessment tools.
2. Mouth mirror.
3. Dental explorer.
4. Mutans streptococci quantification kit.
5. Lactobacilli quantification kit.
6. Saliva buffer capacity test kit.
7. Computer with the Cariogram program installed.

Practice steps

Review caries risk assessment tools

Review different Caries risk assessment tools (Supplemental materials 1 – 3) under the lecturer's instruction.

Students grouping

1. The students are divided into some study groups, each group as a unit consisting of four students.
2. One student plays the role of a child patient, another plays the guardian, and the third student plays the dentist. The fourth student plays the role of a dental assistant and helps to record.

Case assigning

1. The lecturer prepares three typical cases. The caries risk of each case is to be assessed using three different caries risk assessment tools. The serial number is given to each case and the particular caries risk assessment tool.
2. The "patient" is asked to randomly pick a number, then the lecturer or teaching assistant gives all the related information of the case to the "patient".
3. The "patient" and the "guardian" prepare for the role-playing. This whole process should be blinded to the "dentist" and "dentist assistant".

Role-playing

1. The corresponding caries risk assessment form or program is distributed to the group by the

teaching assistant. Please be aware of that the caries-risk assessment forms for different age ranges are to be distributed, the "dentist" has to decide which form to fill in according to the situation of the "patient" later.

2. The "dentist" asks the "patient" or the "guardian" questions from the caries assessment form. The "dentist assistant" helps to record.
3. The "dentist" and "dentist assistant" take an oral examination for the "patient" and record.
4. The "dentist" performs a series of chair-side tests including saliva buffer capacity test (Figure 2 - 1) and/or microbiological examination (Figure 2 - 2) following the provided protocols of corresponding kits.
5. The "dentist" collects all the information of the "patient" and fills in the carries-risk assessment form or gives scores in the "Cariogram".
6. The "dentist" assesses the overall caries risk of the "patient" for the particular case based on the assigned caries risk assessment tool.
7. The "dentist" gives the oral health instructions based on the caries risk of the "patient". The "dentist assistant" need to write down the key points of the oral health instructions given by the "dentist".

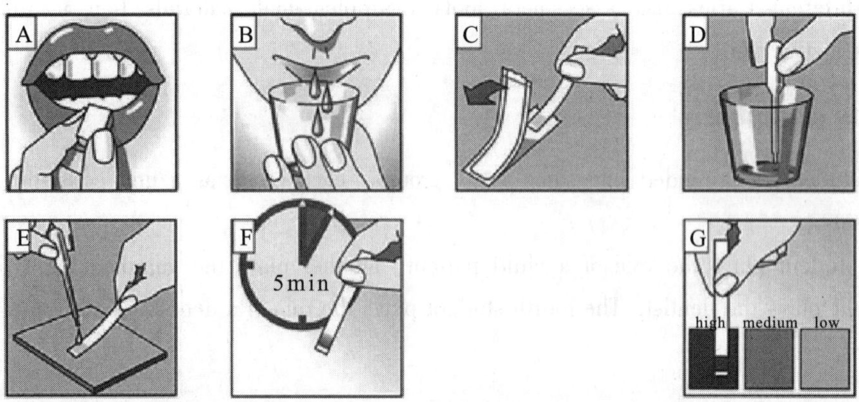

Figure 2 - 1 Step-by-step procedures of saliva buffer capacity test.

A. Stimulate salivation by having your patient chew a paraffin pellet. B. Collect the saliva in a calibrated container. C. Carefully remove the buffer test strip from the packaging without touching the yellow test field. D. Use a pipette to collect a small amount of saliva. E. Place the testing strip on an absorbent paper and wet the entire yellow test field with saliva. F. Wait exactly five minutes of reaction time. G. Compare the color of the testing field with color samples and determine the buffer capacity of saliva.

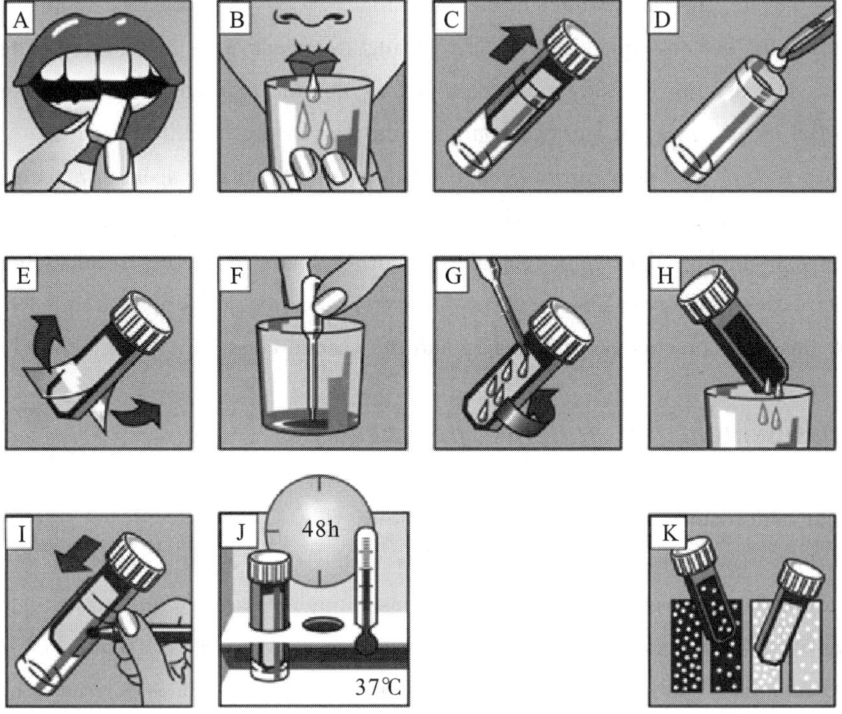

Figure 2 －2　Step-by-step procedures of microbiological examination

A. Stimulate salivation by having your patient chew a paraffin pellet. B. Collect the saliva in a calibrated container. C. Remove the agar carrier from the test vial. D. Place a $NaHCO_3$-tablet at the bottom of the vial. E. Remove the protective foils from the two agar surfaces. Do not touch the agar. F. Use a pipette to collect a small amount of saliva. G. Thoroughly wet both agar surfaces with saliva using a pipette. H. Allow excess saliva to drip off. Slide the agar carrier back into the vial and close the vial tightly. I. Note the name of the patient and the date on the vial. J. Place the test vial upright in the incubator and incubate at 37℃ for 48 hours. K. Compare the density of the mutans streptococci and lactobacilli colonies with the corresponding evaluation pictures in the enclosed model chart.

Make a summary

1. After the role-playing, the "dental assistant" briefly summarizes the information of the case, and collects the recording materials and submits them to the lecturer or the teaching assistant.
2. The lecturer or the teaching assistant judges the performance of each group and gives comments.

Notes

1. When collecting the saliva for saliva buffer capacity test or microbiological examination, collect the saliva over a defined period of five minutes and take this opportunity to measure

the salivation rate (ml saliva/min) at the same time.

2. Do not use the bacteria quantification kit during treatment with antibiotics. After such treatment, at least two weeks should pass before the kit is used. After the use of an antibacterial mouth rinse, at least 12 hours should pass before the kit is used.
3. Before disposing of used agar carriers, disinfect them with a suitable agent or autoclave them in an autoclaving bag.
4. Since the microbiological examination takes about 48 hours to get the results, the whole process of caries risk assessment needs two classes at least two days apart from each other. The first class may practice steps 1 to 10, and the second class may finish steps 11 to 15.

Process assessment for students' practice

1. The overall performance of the student in the role-playing.
2. In-class quiz. The lecturer presents five cases to the class using PowerPoint slides and assigns the caries risk assessment tool for each case. Students are required to write down the judgment of the caries risk level based on the assigned caries risk assessment tool for each case in 5 minutes. The lecturer judges whether the student's answer is correct or not, and gives the class feedbacks.

Supplemental materials

1. Supplemental materials: caries-risk assessment tool (CAT). (Table 2 - 1, Table 2 - 2, Table 2 - 3)

Table 2 - 1 Caries-risk assessment form for 0 - 5 years olds (For dental providers)

Factors	High risk	Moderate risk	Low risk
Biological			
Mother/primary caregiver has active caries	Yes		
Parent/caregiver has low socioeconomic status	Yes		
Child has > 3 between meal sugar-containing snacks or beverages per day	Yes		
Child is put to bed with a bottle containing natural or added sugar	Yes		
Child has special care needs		Yes	
Child is a recent immigrant		Yes	
Protective			

(*to be continued*)

(*Continued*)

Factors	High risk	Moderate risk	Low risk
Child receives optimally-fluoridated drinking water or fluoride supplements			Yes
Child has teeth brushed daily with fluoridated toothpaste			Yes
Child receives topical fluoride from health professional			Yes
Child has dental home/regular dental care			Yes
Clinical findings			
Child has >1 decayed/missing/filled surfaces	Yes		
Child has active white spot lesions or enamel defects	Yes		
Child has elevated mutans streptococci levels	Yes		
Patient has plaque on teeth		Yes	
Circling those conditions that apply to a specific patient helps the practitioner and parent understand the factors that contribute to or protect from caries. Risk assessment categorization of low, moderate, or high is based on preponderance of factors for the individual. However, clinical judgment may justify the use of one factor (i. e., frequent exposure to sugar-containing snacks or beverages, more than one DMFS) in determining overall risk. **Overall assessment of the dental caries risk: High□ Moderate□ Low□**			

Ref. American Academy of Pediatric Dentistry. Guideline on caries-risk assessment and management of infants, children, and adolescents [J]. Pediatric dentistry, 2013, 35 (5): E157 - 164.

Table 2 - 2 Caries-risk assessment form for ≥6 years olds (for dental providers)

Factors	High risk	Moderate risk	Low risk
Biological			
Patient is of low socioeconomic status	Yes		
Patient has >3 between meal sugar-containing snacks or beverages per day	Yes		
Patient has special care needs		Yes	
Patient is a recent immigrant		Yes	
Protective			
Patient receives optimally-fluoridated drinking water			Yes
Patient brushed teeth daily with fluoridated toothpaste			Yes
Patient receives topical fluoride from health professional			Yes
Patient receives additional home measures (i. e., xylitol, MI paste, antimicrobial)			Yes
Patient has dental home/regular dental care			Yes

(*to be continued*)

(*Continued*)

Factors	High risk	Moderate risk	Low risk
Clinical findings			
Patient has >1 interproximal lesions	Yes		
Patient has active white spot lesions or enamel defects	Yes		
Patient has low salivary flow	Yes		
Patient has defective restorations		Yes	
Patient wearing an intraoral appliance		Yes	
Circling those conditions that apply to a specific patient helps the practitioner and parent understand the factors that contribute to or protect from caries. Risk assessment categorization of low, moderate, or high is based on preponderance of factors for the individual. However, clinical judgment may justify the use of one factor (i. e., frequent exposure to sugar-containing snacks or beverages, more than one dmfs) in determining overall risk. **Overall assessment of the dental caries risk: High□ Moderate□ Low□**			

Ref. American Academy of Pediatric Dentistry. Guideline on caries-risk assessment and management of infants, children, and adolescents [J]. Pediatric Dentistry, 2013, 35 (5): E157 - 164.

Table 2 - 3 Example of a caries management protocol for children 6-year-old or younger

Risk category	Diagnostics	Fluoride	Diet	Sealants	Restorative
Low risk	· Recall every 6 to 12 months · Radiographs every 12 to 24 months	Twice daily brushing with fluoridated toothpaste $^{\mu}$	No	Yes	Surveillance $^{\alpha}$
Moderate risk Patient/ parent engaged	· Recall every 6 months · Radiographs every 6 to 24 months	· Twice daily brushing with fluoridated toothpaste $^{\mu}$ · Fluoride supplements $^{\delta}$ · Professional topical treatment every 6 months	Counseling	Yes	· Active surveillance of incipient lesions $^{\varepsilon}$ · Restoration of caviated or enlarging lesions
Moderate risk Patient/parent not engaged	· Recall every 6 months · Radiographs every 6 to 12 months	· Twice daily brushing with fluoridated toothpaste $^{\mu}$ · Professional topical treatment every 6 months	Counseling with limited expectations	Yes	· Active surveillance of incipient lesions $^{\varepsilon}$ · Restoration of caviated or enlarging lesions

(*to be continued*)

(*Continued*)

Risk Category	Diagnostics	Fluoride	Diet	Sealants	Restorative
High risk Patient/ parent engaged	· Recall every 3 months · Radiographs every 6 months	· Brushing with 0.5 percent fluoride · Fluoride supplements[δ] · Professional topical treatment every three months	· Counseling · Xylitol	Yes	· Active surveillance of incipient lesions[ε] · Restoration of caviated or enlarging lesions
High risk Patient/ parent not engaged	· Recall every 3 months · Radiographs every 6 months	· Brushing with 0.5 percent fluoride · Professional topical treatment every 3 months	· Counseling with limited expectations · Xylitol	Yes	· Restore incipient, caviated, or enlarging lesions

α, salivary mutans streptococci bacterial levels; φ, interim therapeutic restoration; γ, parental supervision of a "pea-sized" amount of tooth paste; β, parental supervision of a "smear" amount of toothpaste; λ, indicated for teeth with deep fissure anatomy or developmental defects; χ, periodic monitoring for signs of caries progression; δ, need to consider fluoride levels in drinking water; ε, careful monitoring of caries progression and prevention program; μ, less concern about the quantity of toothpaste.

Ref. American Academy of Pediatric Dentistry. Guideline on caries-risk assessment and management of infants, children, and adolescents [J]. Pediatric dentistry, 2013, 35 (5): E157 - 164.

2. Supplemental material 2: caries management by risk assessment (CAMBRA) (Table 2 - 4 to Table 2 - 6)

Table 2 - 4 CAMBRA for dental providers (0 - 5) assessment tool

Caries risk assessment form for age 0 to 5

Patient name: ____________ I. D. #__________ Age __________ Date __________

Initial/base line exam date ______________ Caries recall date ______________

Respond to each question in sections 1, 2, 3 and 4 with a check mark in the "Yes" or "No" column	Yes	No	Notes
1. Caries risk indicators—patient interview **			
(a) Mother or primary caregivers has had active dental decay in the past 12 months			
(b) Child has recent dental restorations [see 5 (b) below]			
(c) Patient and/or caregiver has low SES (socioeconomic status) and/or low health literacy			
(d) Child has developmental problems			
(e) No dental home/episodic dental care			
2. Caries risk factors (biological) —parent interview **			
(a) Child has frequent (greater than three times daily) between-meal snacks of sugars/cooked starch/sugared beverages			

(*to be continued*)

(*Continued*)

Respond to each question in sections 1, 2, 3 and 4 with a check mark in the "Yes" or "No" column	Yes	No	Notes
(b) Child has saliva-reducing factors present, including: · Medications (i. e. Some for asthma or hyperactivity) · Medical (cancer treatment) or genetic factors			
(c) Child continually uses bottle-contains fluids other than water			
(d) Child sleeps with a bottle or nurses on demand			
3. Protective factors (nonbiological) —parent interview			
(a) Mother/caregiver decay-free last three years			
(b) Child has a dental home and regular dental care			
4. Protective factors (biological) —parent interview			
(a) Child lives in a fluoridated community or takes fluoride supplements by slowly dissolving or as chewable tablets			
(b) Child's teeth are cleaned with fluoridated toothpaste (pea-size) daily			
(c) Mother/caregiver chews/sucks xylitol chewing gum/lozenges 2 – 4x daily			
5. Caries risk indicators/factors—clinical examination of child **			
(a) Obvious white spots, decalcification, or obvious decay present on the child's teeth			
(b) Restorations placed in the last two years in/on child's teeth			
(c) Plaque is obvious on the child's teeth and/or gums bleed easily			
(d) Child has dental or orthodontic appliances present, fixed or removable: i. e., braces, space maintainers, obturator			
(e) Risk Factor: Visually inadequate saliva flow-dry mouth			
** **If yes to any one of 1 (a), 1 (b), 5 (a), or any two in categories 1, 2, 5, consider performing bacterial culture on mother or caregiver and child. Use this as a base line to follow results of antibacterial intervention**	**parent/ care giver** **Date:**		**Child** **Date:**
(a) Mutans streptococci (Indicate bacteria level: high, medium, low)			
(b) Lactobacillus species (Indicate bacteria level: high, medium, low)			
Child's overall caries risk status: (CIRCLE) Extreme	**Low**	**Moderate**	**High**
Recommendations given: Yes ______ No ______ Date given ______ Date follow up ______			
SELF-MANAGEMENT GOALS 1) ______ 2) ______ Practitioner signature ______ Date ______			

Ref. Ramos-Gomez FJ, et al. Caries risk assessment appropriate for the age 1 visit (infants and toddlers) [J]. Journal of the california dental association, 2007, 35 (10): 687 – 702.

Table 2 – 5 CAMBRA treatment guidelines (0 – 5 years)

Caries management by risk assessment (CAMBRA) clinical guidelines for patients 0 – 5 years

Risk level	Saliva test	Antibacterials	Fluoride	Frequency of radiographs	Frequency of periodic oral exams (POE)	**** Xylitol and/or baking soda	Sealants ***	Existing lesions
Low risk	Optional (Bsae line)	Not required or if saliva test was performed; treat main caregiver accordingly	Not required	After age 2: Bitewing radiographs every 18 – 24 months	Every 6 – 12 months to re-evaluate caries risk AND ANTICIPATORY GUIDANCE **		Optional	
Moderate risk	Recommended	Not required or if saliva test was performed; treat main caregiver accordingly	OTC fluoride-containing toothpaste twice daily (a pea-size amount) Sodium fluoride treatment gels rinses	After age 2: Bitewing radiographs every 12 – 18 months	Every 6 months to re-evaluate caries risk and anticipatory guidance	Xylitol gum or lozenges. Two sticks of gum or two mints four times daily for the caregiver Xylitol food, spray, or drinks for the child	Sealants for deep pits and fissures after two years of age. High fluoride conventional glass ionomer is recommended	Lesions that do not penetrate the DEJ and are not cavitated should be treated with fluoride toothpaste and fluoride varnish
High risk *	Required	Chlorhexidine 0.12% 10 ml rinse for main caregiver of the infant or child for one week each month. Bacterial test every caries recall. Health provider might brush infant's teeth with CHX	Fluoride varnish at initial visit and caries recall exams OTC fluoride-containing toothpaste and calcium phosphates paste combination twice daily Sodium fluoride treatment gel/rinses	After age 2; Two size #2 occlusal films and 2 bitewing radiographs every 6 – 12 months or until no cavitated lesions are evident	Every 3 months to re-evaluate caries risk and apply fluoride varnish and anticipatory guidance	Xylitol gum or lozenges Two sticks of gum or two mints four times daily for the caregiver Xylitol food, spray, or drinks for the child	Sealants for deep pits and fissures after two years of age. High fluoride conventional glass ionomer is recommended	Lesions that do not penetrate the DEJ and are not cavitated should be treated with fluoride toothpaste and fluoride varnish ART might be recommended

(*to be continued*)

(*Continued*)

Risk level	Saliva test	Antibacterials	Fluoride	Frequency of radiographs	Frequency of periodic oral exams (POE)	* * * * Xylitol and/or baking soda	Sealants * * *	Existing lesions
Extreme risk *	Required	Chlorhexidine 0.12% 10 ml rinse for one minute daily at bedtime for two weeks each month. Bacterial test at every caries recall Health provider might brush infant's teeth with CHX	Fluoride varnish at initial visit, each caries recall and after prophylaxis or recall exams OTC fluoride-containing toothpaste combination twice daily Sodium fluoride treatment gel/rinses	After age 2; Two size #2 occlusal films and 2 bitewing radiographs every 6 months or until no cavitated lesions are evident	Every 1 – 3 months to re-evaluate caries risk and apply fluoride varnish and anticipatory guidance	Xylitol gum or lozenges Two sticks of gum or two mints four times daily for the caregiver Xylitol food, spray, or drinks	Sealants for deep pits and fissures after two years of age. High fluoride conventional glass ionomer is recommended	Holding care with glass ionomer materials until caries progression is controlled (ART) Fluoride varnish and anticipatory guidance/self-management goals

* Pediatric patients with one (or more) cavitated lesion(s) are high-risk patients.
* Pediatric patients with one (or more) cavitated lesion(s) and hyposalivary or special needs are extreme-risk patients.
* Pediatric patients with daily medication such as inhalers or behavioral issues will have diminished salivary function.
* * Anticipatory guidance – "Appropriate discussion and counseling should be an integral part of each visit for care", AAPD.
* * * ICDAS protocol presented by Jenson et al. this issue may be helpful on sealant decisions.
* * * * Xylitol is not good for pets (especially dogs).
For all risk levels: Pediatric patients, through their caregiver, must maintain good oral hygiene and a diet low in frequency of fermentable carbohydrates.
Patients with appliances (RPDs, orthodontics) require excellent oral hygiene together with intensive fluoride therapy. Fluoride gel to be placed in removable appliance.

Ref. Ramos-Gomez FJ, Crall J, Gansky SA, et al. Caries risk assessment appropriate for the age 1 visit (infants and toddlers) [J]. Journal of the California Dental Association, 2007, 35(10): 687 – 702.

Table 2-6 CAMBRA for dental providers (age 6 and over) assessment tool

Caries risk assessment form—children age 6 and over/adults

Patient name: ________________ Chart#: ________________ Date: ________________

Assessment date: Is this (please circle) base line or recall

Disease indicators (Any one "Yes" signifies likely "High Risk" and to do a bacteria test **)	**Yes = CIRCLE**	**Yes = CIRCLE**	**Yes = CIRCLE**
Visible cavities or radiographic penetration of the dentin	Yes		
Radiographic approximal lesions (not in dentin)	Yes		
White spots on smooth surfaces	Yes		
Restorations last 3 years	Yes		
Risk factors (biological predisposing factors)		Yes	
MS and LB both medium or high (by culture **)		Yes	
Visible heavy plaque on teeth		Yes	
Frequent snack (>3 × daily between meals)		Yes	
Deep pits and fissures		Yes	
Recreational drug use		Yes	
Inadequate saliva flow by observation or measurement (** If measured, note the flow rate below)		Yes	
Saliva reducing factors (medications/radiation/systemic)		Yes	
Exposed roots		Yes	
Orthodontic appliances		Yes	
Protective factors			
Lives/work/school fluoridated community			Yes
Fluoride toothpaste at least once daily			Yes
Fluoride toothpaste at least 2 × daily			Yes
Fluoride mouth rinse (0.05% NaF) daily			Yes
5000 ppm① F fluoride toothpaste daily			Yes
Fluoride varnish in last 6 months			Yes
Office F topical in last 6 months			Yes
Chlorhexidine prescribed/used one week each of last 6 months			Yes
Xylitol gum/lozenges 4 × daily last 6 months			Yes
Calcium and phosphate paste during last 6 months			Yes

(to be continued)

① 注: ppm $=1\times10^{-6}$

(*Continued*)

Disease Indicators (Any one "Yes" signifies likely "High Risk" and to do a bacteria test **)	**Yes = CIRCLE**	**Yes = CIRCLE**	**Yes = CIRCLE**
Adequate saliva flow (>1ml/min stimulated)			Yes
** Bacteria/Saliva Test Results: MS: LB: Flow Rate: ml/min. Date:			
VISUALIZE CARIES BALANCE (Use circled indicators/factors above) (EXTREME RISK = HIGH RISK + SEVERE SALIVARY GLAND HYPOFUNCTION) CARIES RISK ASSESSMENT (CIRCLE): EXTREME HIGH MODERATE LOW Doctor signature/#: __________ Date: __________			

Ref. Featherstone JDB, Domejean-Orliaguet S, et al. Caries risk assessment in practice for age 6 through adult [J]. Journal of the California Dental Association, 2007, 35 (10): 703-707, 710-713.

Table 2 – 7　CAMBRA treatment guidelines (age 6 and older)

Clinical guidelines for patients age 6 and older

Risk level ### ***	Frequency of radiographs	Frequency of caries recall exams	Saliva test (saliva flow & bacterial culture)	Antibacterials chlorhexidine xylitol ****	Fluoride	pH Control	Calcium phosphate topical supplements	Sealants (resin-based or glass ionomer)
Low risk	Bitewing radiographs every 24 – 36 months	Every 6 – 12 months to re-evaluate caries risk	Maybe done as a base line reference for new patients	Per saliva test if done	OTC fluoride-containing toothpaste twice daily, after breakfast and at bedtime, Optional: NaF varnish if excessive root exposure or sensitivity	Not required	Not required Optional: for excessive root exposure or sensitivity	Optional or as per ICDAS sealant protocol
Moderate risk	Bitewing radiographs every 18 – 24 months	Every 4 – 6 months to re-evaluate caries risk	Maybe done as a base line reference for new patients or if there is suspicion of high bacterial challenge and to assess efficacy and patient cooperation	Per saliva test if done Xylitol (6 – 10 grams/day) gum or candies. Two tabs of gum or two candies four times daily	OTC fluoride-containing toothpaste twice daily plus: 0.05% NaF rinse daily. Initially, 1 – 2 appt. of NaF varnish; 1 app at 4 – 6 month recall	Not required	Not required Optional: for excessive root exposure or sensitivity	As per ICDAS sealant protocol
High risk *	Bitewing radiographs every 6 – 18 months or until no cavitated lesions are evident	Every 3 – 4 months to re-evaluate caries risk and apply fluoride varnish	Saliva flow test and bacterial culture initially and at every caries recall appt. to assess efficacy and patient cooperation	Chlorhexidine gluconate 0.12% 10 ml rinse for one minute daily for one week each month. Xylitol 6 – 10 grams/day) gum or candies. Two tabs of gum or two candies four times daily	1.1% NaF toothpaste twice daily instead of regular fluoride toothpaste. Optional: 0.2% NaF rinse daily (1 bottle) then OTC 0.05% NaF rinse 2 × daily. Initially 1 – 3 app. NaF varnish; 1 appt. at 3 – 4 month recall	Not required	Optional: apply calcium/phosphate paste several times daily	As per ICDAS sealant protocol

(*to be continued*)

(*Continued*)

Risk level ### ***	Frequency of radiographs	Frequency of caries recall exams	Saliva test (saliva flow & bacterial culture)	Antibacterials chlorhexidine xylitol ****	Fluoride	pH Control	Calcium phosphate topical supplements	Sealants (resin-based or glass ionomer)
Extreme risk ** (High risk plus dry mouth or special needs)	Bitewing radiographs every 6 months or until no cavitated lesions are evident	Every 3 months to re-evaluate caries risk and apply fluoride varnish	Saliva flow test and bacterial culture initially and at every caries recall appt. to assess efficacy and patient cooperation	Chlorhexidine 0.12% (preferably CHX in water base rinse) 10 ml rinse for one minute daily for one week each month. Xylitol (6 – 10 grams/day) gum or candies. Two tabs of gum or two candies four times daily	1.1% NaF toothpaste twice daily instead of regular fluoride toothpaste. Optional: 0.05% NaF rinse when mouth feels dry, after snacking, breakfast, and lunch. Initially 1 – 3 appt. NaF varnish; 1 app at 3 month recall	Acid-neutralizing rinses as needed if mouth feels dry, after snacking, bedtime and after breakfast. Baking Soda gum as needed	Required: apply calcium/ phosphate paste twice daily	As per ICDAS sealant protocol

* Patients with one (or more) cavitated lesion(s) are high-risk patients.
** Patients with one (or more) cavitated lesion(s) and severe hyposalivation are extreme-risk patients.
*** All restorative work to be done with the minimally invasive philosophy in mind. Existing smooth surface lesions that do not penetrate the DEJ and are not cavitated should be treated chemically, not surgically. For extreme-risk patients, use holding care with glass ionomer materials until caries progression is controlled. Patients with appliances (RPDs, prosthodontics) require excellent oral hygiene together with intensive fluoride therapy e.g., high fluoride toothpaste and fluoride varnish every three months. Where indicated, antibacterial therapy to be done in conjunction with restorative work.
For all risk levels: Patients must maintain good oral hygiene and a diet low in frequency of fermentable carbohydrates.
*** Xylitol is not good for pets (especially dogs)

Ref. Jenson L, Budenz AW, Featherstone JDB, et al. Clinical protocols for caries management by risk assessment [J]. Journal of the California Dental Association. 2007, 35(10): 714 – 723.

3. Supplemental material 3: Cariogram. (Table 2-8, Figure 2-1)

Table 2-8 Caries related factors and the data needed to create a Cariogram

Factors*	Comment	Info/data needed
Caries experience	Past caries experience, including cavities, fillings and missing teeth because of caries. Several new cavities definitely appearing during preceding year should give a high score even if number of fillings is low	DMFT, DMFS, new caries experience in the past 1 year
Related disease	General disease or conditions associated with dental caries	Medical history, medications
Diet, contents	Estimation of the cariogenicity of the food, in particular sugar contents	Diet history, lactobacillus test count
Diet, frequency	Estimation of number of meals and snacks per day, mean for "normal days"	Questionnaire results, 24h recall or dietary recall (3 days)
Plaque amount	Estimation of hygiene, for example according to Silness-Löe Plaque Index (PI). Crowded teeth leading to difficulties in removing plaque interproximally should be taken into account	Plaque index
Mutans streptococci	Estimation of levels of mutans streptococci (*Streptococcus mutans*, *Sretptococcus sobrinus*) in saliva, for example using Strip mutans test	Strip mutans test or other laboratory tests giving comparable results
Fluoride programme	Estimation of to what extent fluoride is available in the oral cavity over the coming period of time	Fluoride exposure, interview patient
Saliva secretion	Estimation of amount of saliva, for example using paraffin-stimulated secretion and expressing results as milliliter saliva per minute	Stimulated saliva test—secretion rate
Saliva buffer capacity	Estimation of capacity of saliva to buffer acids, for example using Dentobuff test	Dentobuff test or other laboratory tests giving comparable results

* For each factor, the examiner has to gather information by interviewing and examining the patient, including some saliva tests. The information is then given a score of a scale ranging from 0 to 3 (0-2 for some factors) according to predetermined criteria. The score "0" is the most favorable value and the maximum score "3" (or "2") indicates a high, unfavorable risk value.

Ref. Bratthall D, Hänsel Petersson G, et al. Cariogram—a multifactorial risk assessment model for a multifactorial disease [J]. Community Dentistry and Oral Epidemiology, 2005, 33(4): 256-264.

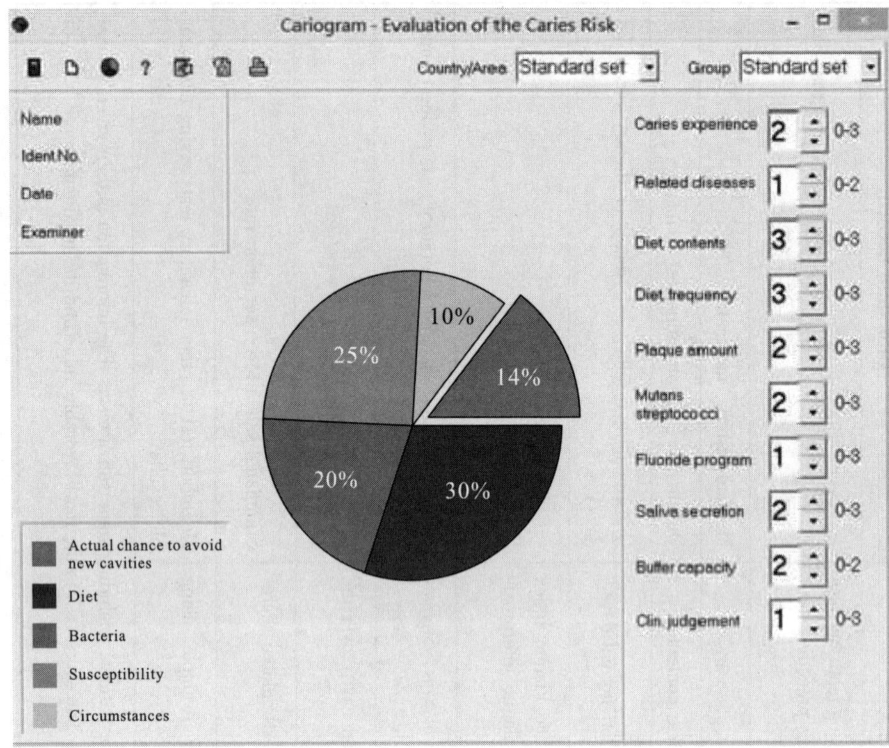

Figure 2 -1. Example of a Cariogram indicating high caries risk with the "chance of avoiding caries (new cavities)" estimated to only 14%.

References

[1] American Academy of Pediatric Dentistry. Guideline on caries-risk assessment and management of infants, children, and adolescents [J]. Pediatric Dentistry, 2013, 35 (5): E157 -164.

[2] Ramos-Gomez FJ, Crall J, Gansky SA, et al. Caries risk assessment appropriate for the age 1 visit (infants and toddlers) [J]. Journal of the California Dental Association, 2007, 35 (10): 687 -702.

[3] Featherstone JDB, Domejean-Orliaguet S, Jenson L, et al. Caries risk assessment in practice for age 6 through adult [J]. Journal of the California Dental Association, 2007, 35 (10): 703 -707, 710 -713.

[4] Jenson L, Budenz AW, Featherstone JDB, et al. Clinical protocols for caries management by risk assessment [J]. Journal of the California Dental Association, 2007, 35 (10): 714 -723.

[5] Bratthall D, Hänsel Petersson G. Cariogram—a multifactorial risk assessment model for a multifactorial disease [J]. Community Dentistry and Oral Epidemiology, 2005, 33 (4): 256 -264.

CHAPTER 3

LOCAL ANESTHESIA TECHNIQUES IN PEDIATAL DENTAL CLINIC

Pain control in pediatric patients with local anesthesia

Profound pain management in pediatric patients with local anesthesia facilitates successful treatment by releasing their anxiety and discomfort during dental treatment procedures. Good operating techniques on local anesthesia in pediatric patients requires understanding to the characteristics of child growth and development, pediatric behavior management, and techniques and pharmacology of local anesthetics. Before any anesthetic administration, a comprehensive medical review and evaluation should be conducted for the selection of anesthetic agents and techniques, which includes but is not limited to potential allergy, body weight and adverse drug interactions, and completion of medical consults as needed.

In general, the techniques employed during local anesthetic procedures on pediatric patients could be categorized in three types: topical, infiltration and nerve block. Topical anesthesia is used to control the discomfort associated with the insertion of the needle into the mucosal membrane. Several disadvantages in the application of this techniques, including the effectiveness of pain management in complicated or prolonged treatment procedures and the taste of anesthetic agents. Both infiltration and nerve block anesthesia necessitate needles and injection techniques in order to establish sound pain control. However, the fear and anticipation of pediatric patients to the discomfort by needle penetration may obstacle the successful application of both techniques. In addition, the complications following local anesthesia may include various local and systemic effects, i. e. masticatory trauma, needle breakage, hematomas and infections.

The indications for administrating local anesthesia in pediatric dental clinic

1. Restorative and surgical operations which may cause pain or discomfort to the pediatric patients, including but not limited to tooth preparation, pulp therapy and tooth extraction.

2. Treatment preparation procedures which may associate with the discomfort or pain.

Introduction to computer-controlled local anesthesia techniques

The simplest and most effective method of reducing pain during dental procedures is local anesthesia. Despite careful anesthetic procedures, dental local anesthesia can still cause pain for various reasons, including soft tissue damage during penetration of the oral mucosa, pressure from the spread of the anesthetic solution, temperature of anesthetic solution, pH of anesthetic solution, and pain from the characteristics of the drug. In addition, the anticipation of receiving a "shot" also tends to increase anxiety of the pediatric patients. Thus, they may exhibit negative behavior before, during and after the injection.

Among all the available methods for pain control during the procedures of local anesthesia for pediatric patients, reducing the injection speed is the most effective method in reducing pain. Unfortunately, controlling and maintaining the amount or speed of injection in actual clinical settings is difficult.

In general, the conventional techniques of local anesthesia delivery can successfully be employed for children in the dental clinic. However, this experience can be overwhelming and disruptive to some children. In recent years, alternative delivery systems of dental anesthesia have been made available. In this section, the computer-controlled local anesthetic delivery system and corresponded operative guideline will be introduced.

Many devices have been introduced that can inject local anesthetics into the tissues at a set speed. Collectively, these "painless anesthetic devices", are termed "computer-controlled local anesthetic delivery" (CCLAD) devices. CCLAD also collectively refers to devices that not only slow and maintain the injection speed, but also maintain a constant speed while taking into account the anatomical characteristics of the tissues being injected. The devices of this type include the Comfort Control™ Syringe (CCS; DENTSPLY, USA), QuickSleeper (Dental HiTec, France) and iCT (Dentium, Seoul, Korea). Among all the CCLAD devices, the most widely known and representative one is the Wand™ (Milestone Scientific, Livingstone, NJ) with STA (single tooth anesthesia) system. In this chapter, we will practice CCLAD via the STA system.

The CCLAD can perform all types of traditional injections that are routinely performed to achieve effective local anesthesia in dentistry. In addition, the CCLAD enables the dentist to perform several new dental injection techniques that were developed in conjunction with this technology. The anterior middle superior alveolar (AMSA), the palatal anterior superior alveolar (P-ASA) and intraligamentary injections are unique dental injections in that they require precise flow-rate and pressure to safely and properly perform. Each of these injections can be used effectively as a primary dental injection when treating pediatric patients.

The objective of lab practice

1. Be familiar with the principle of computer controlled local anesthesia technique: control the flow rate and pressure of the anesthesia during the injection.
2. Be familiar with the basic operations of supra-periosteal infiltration by using the CCLAD.
3. To know the clinical techniques by using CCLAD: Intraligamentary injection, AMSA, P-ASA.
4. To know how to choose the appropriate anesthesia method according to clinical needs.

Materials and instruments

1. CCLAD (the STA system).
2. Handpiece.
3. Local anesthetic (i. e. , articaine hydrochloride).
4. Dental training model.

Practice steps

Introduction of CCLAD (the STA system)

Figure 3 - 1 and Figure 3 - 2 illustrate the computer-controlled local anesthetic delivery devices with STA System, and the operation panel of STA system.

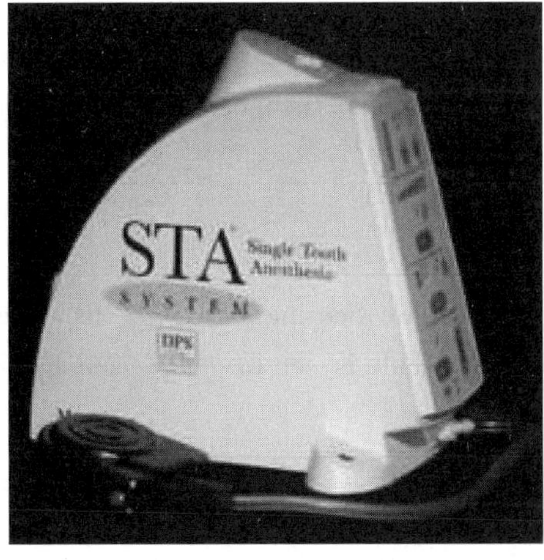

(A) STA system

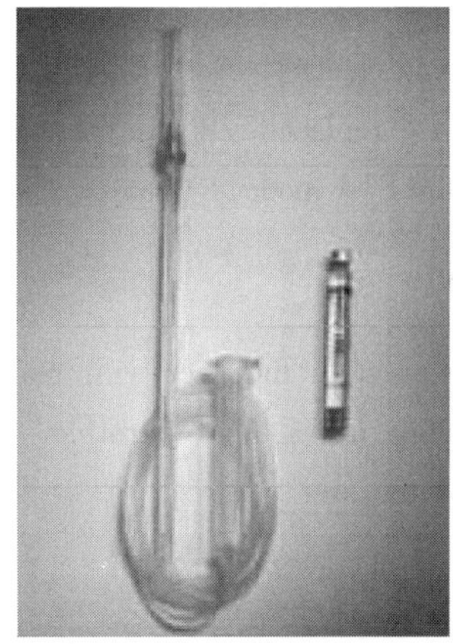

(B) Handpiece and local anesthetic

Figure 3 - 1 Introduction of CCLAD.

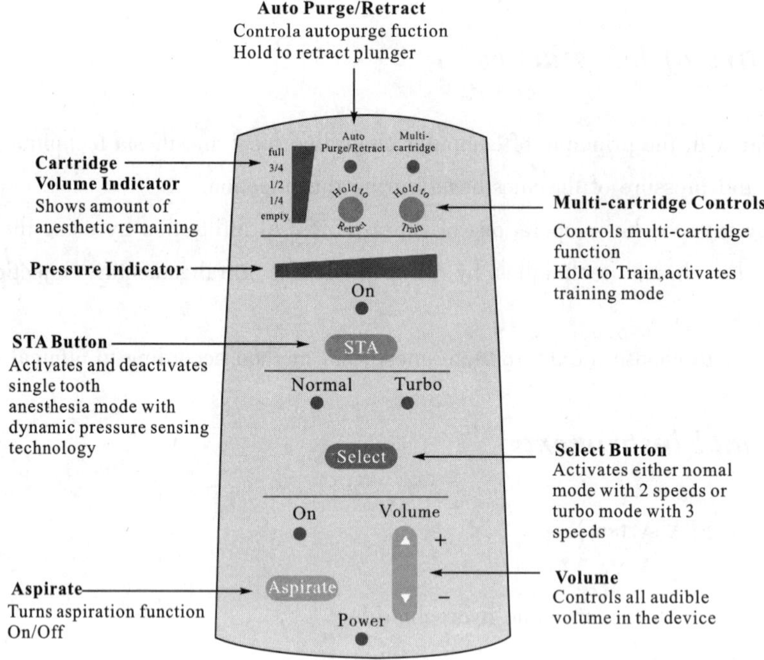

Figure 3 −2 The operation panel of STA system.

Basic modes of operation

The STA system is equipped with three basic modes of operation. They are:

- STA mode, which has a single anesthetic injection flow rate. This mode is activated when the unit is turned on.
- Normal mode, which has 2 anesthetic injection flow rates.
- Turbo mode, which has 3 anesthetic injection flow rates.

The user may change between modes during any procedure and the selection is retained while cartridges are replaced. When the STA system is turned off and then back on, the default setting is the STA mode.

STA mode

STA mode provides the user with real-time Dynamic Pressure Sensing (DPS™) technology while injecting using the ControlFlo™ rate. Aspiration default is set to "On" and can be changed by the user.

Normal mode

The normal mode, the system has 2 flow rates, ControlFlo™ and RapidFlo™. The DPS™ pressure sensing technology is not activated. Aspiration is set to "On" and can be changed to "Off" by the user.

Turbo mode

The Turbo mode provides the user with an additional speed, TurboFlo™; all three speeds are controlled by the foot-control pedal. Aspiration is set to "On" and can be changed to "Off" by the user.

The handpiece placement

Familiarize with the operation of the STA system by practicing with the device before clinical use.

- Turn drive instrument on.
- Remove a needle from the sterile packaging. Maintain sterility.
- Hold the handpiece firmly. Place the needle into the open end of the handpiece and rotate needle. It is critical that the needle is firmly secured to the handpiece.
- Slide the diaphragm end of the cartridge (with a metal band) into the cartridge holder, push cartridge firmly and completely into the holder until you feel the spike penetrates the rubber diaphragm.
- Place open, flange end of cartridge holder into the cartridge holder socket on top of the instrument, and rotate counter-clockwise 1/4 turn.
- After attaching the cartridge holder to the driving instrument, the STA system will automatically purge the air from the tubing and needle. The handpiece is now primed and ready for use.

One-handed needle recapping technique

One-handed needle recapping technique is an essential technique utilizing the STA system, not only offering effectiveness in clinical practice, but also preventing accidental exposure.

- After the needle is attached to the handpiece, place the needle cap into the wand holder on either side of the STA system.
- Hold needle cap firmly with one hand, remove the needle from the cap with the other hand by pulling straight out from the cap. Do not twist (cap remains in the receptacle on the side of the instrument).
- Between injections, lightly set the needle back into the cap. Do not press into the cap. This is a temporary holding dock for the needle.
- When ready to use the handpiece and needle, simply remove the handpiece and needle from the cap. Return the needle to the cap when not in use.
- When the procedure is completed, firmly press the needle into the cap on the side of the STA system, locking the cap back on the needle. When locked in place and keeping your hands behind needle point, remove the cap with the attached needle from the instrument and discard it in an approved manner.

Performing the supraperiosteal infiltration technique

The CCLAD is ideally suited for the administration of supraperiosteal infiltration. The steps for this technique include:

· Holding the handpiece in a pen-like grasp, place the needle near the mucobuccal fold.
· Perform an aspiration pre-test (the aspiration feature is set to the "On" position).
· Initiate the ControlFlo™ (first foot control position) flow rate.
· Slight needle rotation at the moment of mucosa puncture facilitates penetration of the surface tissue.
· Penetrate mucosa with slow, gentle advancement of the needle to create an "anesthetic pathway".
· When the needle reaches the target site, aspiration can be initiated if required (release foot control).
· Aspiration is repeated until negative aspiration is observed.
· When aspiration is negative, initiate the RapidFlo™ (second foot control position) flow rate.
· Monitor the LED panel to determine the volume of anesthetic delivered.
· When the cartridge is emptied (audio and visual signal), reload, purge and continue as required.

Performing the intraligamentary injection technique

The periodontal ligament injection has long been advocated as a rapid, site-specific technique to anesthetize a specific tooth and the adjacent periodontal tissue. Some of the literature suggests that due to the pressure required to administer this injection in the traditional method with a conventional syringe or other mechanical devices, it may be contraindicated in primary teeth and teeth with active periodontal infection or suppuration. The steps for this technique include:

· Verify the instrument is set to "STA-Mode".
· While holding the handpiece in a pen-like grasp, place the needle into the gingival sulcus of the tooth to be anesthetized. Simultaneously, activate the ControlFlo™ flow rate by depressing the foot control. It is important to gently and slowly advance the needle within the sulcus as if it were a periodontal probe.
· Begin injection at the distal site followed by mesial.
· As the pressure increases the visual pressure sensing scale on the front of the instrument, the LED lights will change from orange to yellow to green.
· A drug volume of 0. 5 ml is recommended for single-rooted teeth. A drug volume of 0. 9 ml is recommended for multi-rooted teeth.

Figure 3 – 3 shows details of the intraligamentary injection.

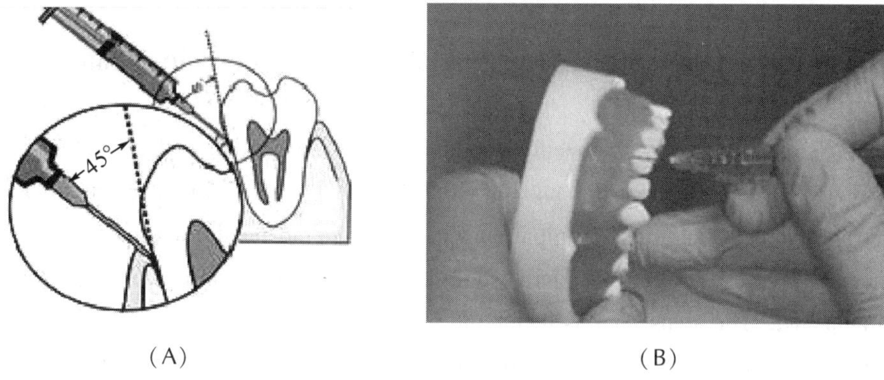

(A) (B)

Figure 3 - 3 Intraligamentary injection illustration.

Performing the anterior middle superior alveolar (AMSA) injection technique

The AMSA is an exciting addition to local anesthesia techniques. It will allow the operator to achieve pulpal anesthesia from the maxillary central incisor through the second premolar including the palatal tissue and mucoperiosteum from a single needle penetration. The lips, face and muscles of expression are not anesthetized with the AMSA resulting in greater patient comfort operatively and postoperatively. The steps for this technique include:

- It is inserted in a position that bisects the premolars and is approximately halfway between the mid-palatine suture and the free gingival margin.
- Pre-puncture: The needle bevel is initially oriented parallel to the palatal tissue. The foot control is depressed slightly to activate the ControlFlo™ flow rate for 8 - 10 beeps prior to slow needle insertion.
- The needle is reoriented to a 45° angle as it is advanced until it contacts the bone. Performing aspiration. Then maintain contact on the bone and deliver the required dosage of 3/4 to 1 cartridge.
- Significant blanching of the palate will be observed.
- Remove the needle slowly and try to avoid any excess anesthetic dripping into the mouth.

Figure 3 - 4 demonstrates the landmark of AMSA injection.

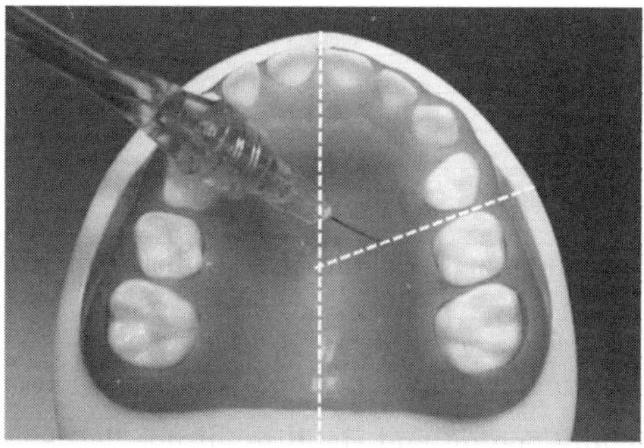

Figure 3 - 4 Landmark of AMSA injection.

Performing the palatal anterior superior alveolar (P-ASA) injection technique

The P-ASA is another modified injection for the anterior maxilla. It will allow the operator to achieve bilateral anesthesia of the maxillary incisors and usually the canines from a single needle penetration. In addition to pulpal anesthesia, profound palatal anesthesia of the gingiva and mucoperiosteum as well as moderate anesthesia of the facial gingiva associated with the teeth is achieved. The steps for this technique include:

- It is inserted adjacent to the incisive papilla.
- Pre-puncture: The needle bevel is initially oriented as parallel to the palatal tissue as possible. The foot control is depressed slightly to activate the ControlFlo™ flow rate for 8 – 10 beeps prior to slow needle insertion. After penetration into the papilla, insertion is continued until significant blanching of the papilla is observed.
- The needle is then reoriented to gain entrance into the nasopalatine canal and advanced very slowly for no more than 1 cm. Maintaining contact on the bony wall of the canal and then aspirate.
- Deliver the required dosage of 3/4 to 1 cartridge. Significant blanching of the palate tissue and often the facial tissue will be observed.
- Remove the needle slowly to avoid excess dripping into the mouth.

Figure 3 – 5 demonstrates landmark of P-ASA injection.

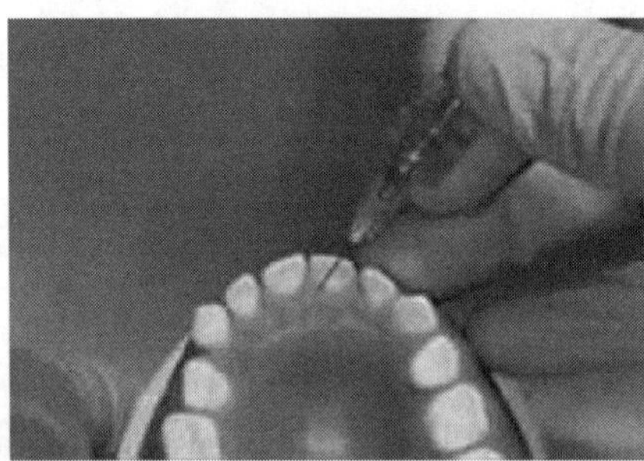

(A) Initiate P-ASA

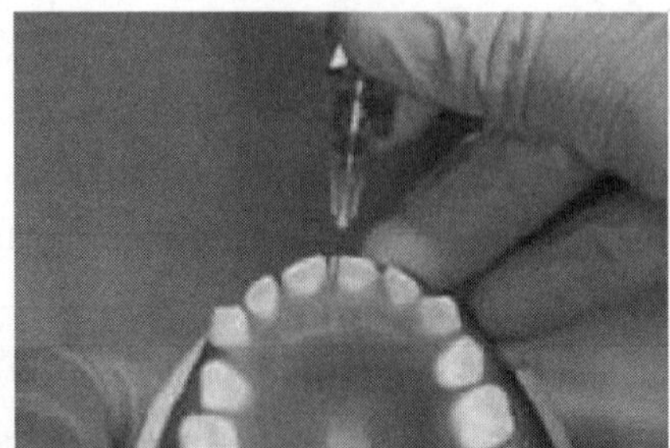

(B) Reorient P-ASA

Figure 3 – 5 Landmark of P-ASA injection.

Tips

1. 30 gauge 1/2 inch needle and 4% Articaine Hydrochloride 1 : 200,000 vasoconstrictors are recommended.
2. Perform aspiration to prevent injection into blood vessels.
3. Use a finger-rest to carefully control and stabilize all needle movements.
4. It is the responsibility of each practitioner to identify, select and administer the proper drug

volume for a given patient. Especially for children, the age, weight and allergic history should be considered.

5. It is very important to choose the appropriate anesthesia method according to clinical needs.

Process assessment for students' practice

The instructor will grade the students' practice according to:

- Proper selection and placement of the handpiece.
- Correct setting of the STA system.
- Proper techniques for preventing occupational exposure.
- Correct operative techniques of the basic operation and listed local anesthetic techniques.

References

[1] The American Academy of Pediatric Dentistry. Use of local anesthesia for pediatric dental patients [J]. Pediatr Dent, 2017, 39 (6): 266 -272.

[2] Malamed SF. Local anesthesia [J]. J Calif Dent Assoc, 1998, 26 (9): 657 -660.

[3] Saloum FS, Baumgartner JC, Marshall G, et al. A clinical comparison of pain perception to the wand and a traditional syringe [J]. Oral Surg, Oral Med, Oral Pathol, Oral Radiol, and Endod, 2000, 89 (6): 691 -695.

[4] Hochman M, Chiarello D, Hochman CB, et al. Computerized local anesthetic delivery vs. traditional syringe technique. Subjective pain response [J]. N Y State Dent J, 1997, 63 (7): 24 -29.

CHAPTER 4

BEHAVIOR MANAGEMENT TECHNIQUES IN PEDIATRIC DENTISTRY

Introduction to behavior management techniques

The process of promoting a child and her/his parents to cooperate with the dentists through the dental appointment has been termed as dental behavior management. In 2003, the American Academy of Pediatric Dentistry (AAPD) introduced this term behavior guidance in its clinical guidelines to emphasize that the goals are not to "deal with" a child's behavior but rather to enhance communication and partner with the child and parent to promote a positive attitude toward oral health care and further good oral health.

The objective of lab practice

1. To master the Frankl behavior rating scale to rate children's cooperative behaviors.
2. To be familiar with non-pharmacologic management of children's behaviors.
3. To know pharmacologic management of children's behaviors.

Materials

Pictures showing different kind of children behavior in pediatric dentistry.

Content for instruction

Frankl behavior rating scale

Frankl behavior rating scale is used to evaluate children's cooperation/behavior. The behavior rating should be recorded in the progress notes for each dental visit. The scoring system ranges from 1 to 4. Table 4 – 1 describes the categories of Frankl behavior rating scale. This score is quite helpful in developing strategies for behavior guidance at future appointments and is essential for treatment planning.

Table 4 – 1 Frankl behavior rating scale

Score rate	Categories of behavior
Rating 1	Definitely negative. Refusal of treatment, forceful crying, fearfulness, or any other overt evidence of extreme negativism
Rating 2	Negative. Reluctance to accept treatment, uncooperativeness, some evidence of negative attitude but not pronounced (sullen, withdrawn)
Rating 3	Positive. Acceptance of treatment; cautious behavior at times; willingness to comply with the dentist, at times with reservation, but follows the dentist's directions cooperatively
Rating 4	Definitely positive. Good rapport with the dentist, interested in dental procedures, laughter, and enjoyment

Information evaluating child's behavior can be gathered from the parent through questions regarding the child's cognitive level, temperament/personality characteristics, anxiety and fear, reaction to strangers, and behavior at previous medical/dental visits, as well as how the parent anticipates the child will respond to future dental treatment. The dentist can evaluate cooperative potential by observation and interacting with the patient. Whether the child is approachable, somewhat shy, or definitely shy and/or withdrawn may influence the success of various communicative techniques. Assessing the child's development, past experiences, and current emotional state allows the dentist to develop a behavior guidance plan to accomplish the necessary oral health care. During the delivery of care, the dentist must remain attentive to the physical and/or emotional indicators of stress. Changes in adaptive behaviors may require alterations to the behavioral treatment plan.

Non-pharmacologic management of children's behaviors

The non-pharmacologic behavior guidance techniques can be used by the dentist and auxiliaries to help children reduce or eliminate fear, learn to cooperate during dental treatment and be willing to return for further dental care.

• Expectations

Children learn helpful behavior in the dental office if they understand what is expected of them. It is the function of the dentist and the auxiliaries to define precisely the helpful behavior that is expected of the child.

• Modeling

A child may model other children he sees in the dental office. It is useful sometimes to allow a new patient, especially a young child, to sit quietly and watch a sibling or another child being treated.

• Pretreatment experience

Help the child learn about dental treatment by showing them around the dental office and communicating appropriately at the child's level of understanding (use euphemisms or word substitutes).

• Association

A very useful aspect of association as a means of guiding behavior is through unlearning unpleasant associations and replacing them with more pleasant associations. This use of association is a reason for arranging the treatment sequence in a way that places the least stressful treatments first and delays the more unpleasant treatments until after the child has been able to make some pleasant associations with dental care.

• Positive reinforcement

Give the child a stimulus that he regards as desirable immediately following the reinforced behavior. The rewards most often used in the dental office are in the form of words of praise, hugs, and other means of demonstrating to the child that he or she has done something that others admire.

• Tell-show-do

Tell the child what is to be done, show the child what is to be done, and then proceed to do exactly what the child has been led to expect. The information used in "tell, show, do" varies according to the developmental level of the child and his previous experiences.

• Voice control

Influence children's behavior by changing the speed, volume or tone of the voice. How it is said is more important than what is said because the dentist is attempting to influence behavior directly, not through understanding.

• In-office dental treatment with restraint

If a child is uncooperative it can be possible to provide dental care using physical restraints to control body movement. Restraints might include holding child's hands and arms, legs, head, the use of a mouth prop, or full-body restraint using a papoose board or velcro straps. Using child restraints has the risk of causing skin irritation and may be strongly resisted by your child. The amount of treatment that can be provided at any one visit is limited and children with extensive treatment needs will require several visits.

Pharmacologic management of patient behavior

Most children can be managed effectively using the non-pharmacologic management techniques. Such techniques should form the foundation for all the management activities provided by the dentist. However, some children cannot cooperate due to a history of past traumatic medical/dental experiences, high anxiety levels with minimal coping skills, lack of psychological or emotional maturity and/or mental, physical, or medical disability. They require more advanced techniques to control body movements and decrease anxiety. Pharmacologic management is a broad term that describes the use of drugs to manage the behavior of pediatric patients undergoing dental procedures, including sedation and general anesthesia.

- **Nitrous oxide-oxygen inhalation sedation**

Nitrous oxide inhalation sedation is the method of behavioral management in potentially cooperative children > 3 years of age. It is also useful in children with a limited attention span who have trouble sitting still for more than a few minutes, those with a strong gag reflex that interferes with dental treatment and in children who have uncontrolled movements as a result of a neurological disorder.

- **Oral sedation**

It works best for children 2 to $4\frac{1}{2}$ years of age who need only one or two appointments to complete their treatment needs.

- **Intravenous sedation**

The intravenous route of administration shares most of the desirable pharmacokinetic and pharmacodynamics features of inhalational anesthetics, but it is often difficult to achieve sustained moderate sedation through the intravenous route in the pediatric patient. This modality is best suited to older children and adolescents for a combination of behavioral, pharmacologic, and practical reasons.

- **General anesthesia**

Sometimes the sedation will not be effective and we may recommend that the child be treated under general anesthesia. All their dental treatment needs can be completed in one visit.

Practice steps

1. The instructor describes the performance of patients and shows it by pictures. Students are

asked to rate the cooperative behavior and record it on paper according to Frankl behavior rating scale. Their answers are gathered and the instructor will give scores based on their answers.

2. Divide students into groups and different students play different roles, such as "dentist," "nurse," "parent" or "patient." Simulate the clinic situation of nonpharmacologic management of children's behaviors by the practice of role-playing.
   - Divide students into groups beforehand and four in one group. Specific tasks are randomly assigned to each group to perform one type of nonpharmacologic management of children's behaviors before the class.
   - One representative of each group explains their understanding of the nonpharmacologic management that they are trying to show.
   - Introduce everyone's role in the group. Who plays the patient? Who plays the dentist? Who plays the nurse? Who plays the parent?
   - Give the specific clinic situation they are facing. The following information should be included but not limited to the following items.

How old is the patient?
Who accompany the patient into the clinic?
What is the chief complaint of the child?
Does the patient come to the clinic for the first time or has he/she visited the dentist several times?
What treatment was given and how did the patient perform during the last dental visit?
What is the result of the clinical examination?
What is the score of children's cooperative behavior by Frankl behavior rating scale?
What kind of treatment will be given?

   - The instructor makes comments on the whole play and each role at the end of the show. Students in other groups are encouraged to express their comments.
   - Scores are given by the instructor according to their performance and feedback given by other groups.

Process assessment for students' practice

1. Accurate assessment of patient behavior by Frankl behavior rating scale.
2. Proper application of non-pharmacologic management according to patient behavior.

Tips

1. Effective pain control: the best management efforts can be undermined by inadequate

anesthesia. Local anesthesia and pain control for the child is one of the most important aspects of child behavior guidance in the dental office during dental procedures.

2. The dentist should choose the agent and technique that best fit the patient type as well as the nature of what needs to be accomplished.
3. A thorough review of the medical history, along with a focused physical assessment, is required to determine whether a patient is a good candidate for sedation or general anesthesia.
4. Informed consent: the parent or legal guardian must consent to the use of sedation and general anesthesia for the child. These individuals are entitled to receive complete information regarding the reasonably foreseeable risks and the benefits associated with the particular technique(s) and agents being used, as well as any alternative methods available.

References

Dean JA, Jones JE, Walker Vinson LA. McDonald and Avery's dentistry for the child and adolescent [M]. 10th ed. St. Louis: Elsevier, 2016.

CHAPTER 5

PREVENTIVE RESIN RESTORATION FOR IMMATURE PERMANENT MOLARS

Introduction to preventive resin restoration

The preventive resin restoration(PRR) is an alternative procedure for restoring primary teeth and immature permanent teeth that require only minimal tooth preparation for caries removal but also have adjacent susceptible fissures. A resin restoration was placed for the prepared cavity, and the adjacent pits and fissures were sealed at the same time

PRR is particularly applicable for young patients with recently erupted teeth and minimally carious pits and fissures. This preparation requires a meticulous technique that involves more time than the preparation for the traditional occlusal amalgam restoration. This type of restoration was advocated for carefully selected non-stress-bearing areas to minimize anatomic wear. Teeth that are suitable for PRR are those that demonstrate small, discrete regions of decay, often limited to a single pit. As with sealants, the ability to isolate the tooth and keep it dry throughout the procedure is the most important indication.

It has been reported 79% retention of PRR in permanent molars after 9 years and concluded that the PRR was a successful conservative alternative to the treatment of minimal occlusal caries. Although long-term retention studies of PRR in primary teeth are lacking, with retention rates of PRR and sealants in permanent teeth being very similar, it is reasonable to believe that retention rates of PRR in primary teeth would also be similar to sealant rates.

Indications

The teeth with small class Ⅰ cavities and adjacent susceptible pits and fissures of cooperative children.

The objective of lab practice

1. To master the indication of PRR.

2. To know the rationale of PRR.
3. To be familiar with the procedures of PRR.

Materials and instruments

1. For tooth cleaning: low-speed handpiece, small dental brush or bristle brush (rubber cup) and non-fluoridated toothpaste (polishing paste) [Figure 5 - 1 (A) and (B)].
2. For caries removal: high-speed handpiece, small-particle diamond burs or a laser system (if available) [Figure 5 - 1 (A)].
3. For isolation: rubber dam (if available) or cotton rolls [Figure 5 - 1 (C) and (D)].
4. 37% phosphoric acid solution, composite resin, bonding agents, visible light-cured sealant, visible curing light, articulating paper [Figure 5 - 1 (E) and (F)].

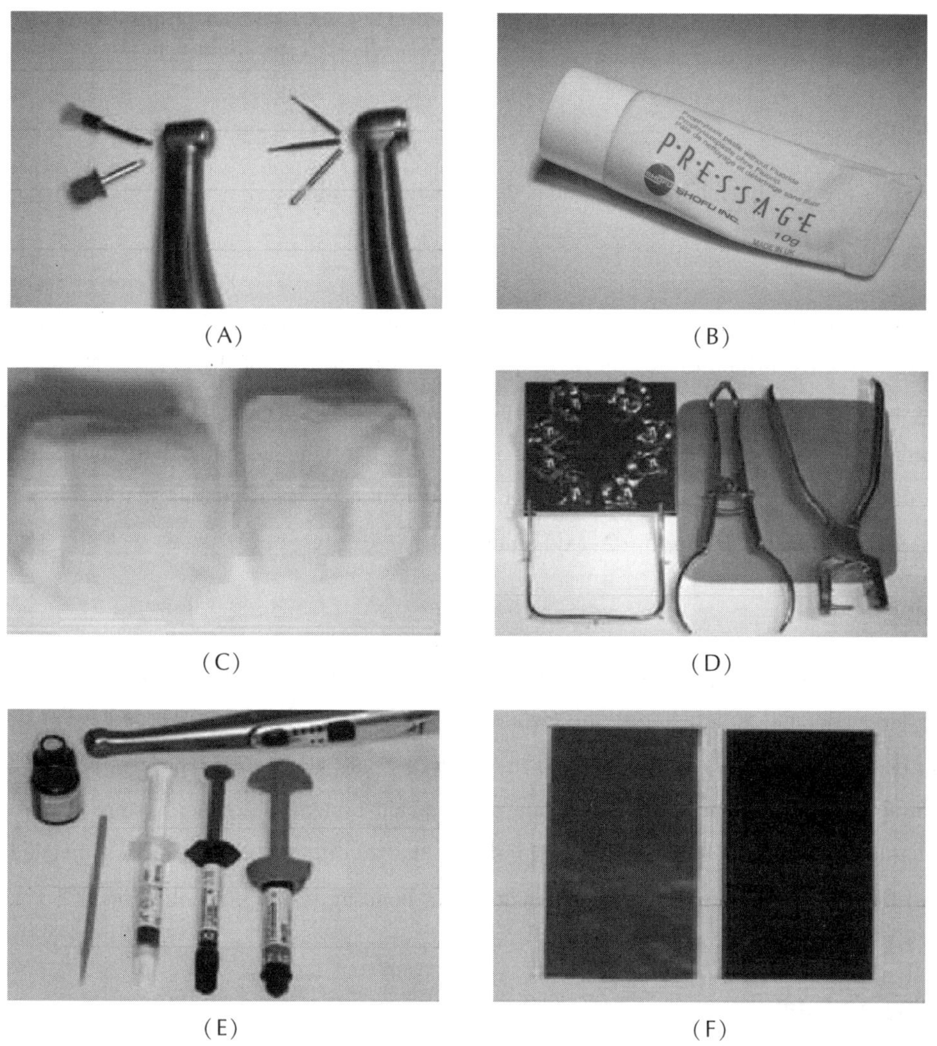

Figure 5 - 1 Materials and instruments.

Practice steps

Cleaning

Use a rotating dry bristle brush with toothpaste to clean the dental plaque, debris or pigments on the teeth. Adequate retention of the sealant requires that the pits and fissures be clean and free of excess moisture [Figure 5 - 2 (A)].

Identification of caries

Tactile probing the tooth surface with a round-end explore, visual examination of a dry occlusal tooth surface white spot lesion or dark stains to identify the incipient and latent caries. In the clinic, diagnostic tools, like quantitative light fluorescence (QLF) can be used [Figure 5 - 2 (B)].

Isolation

Cotton rolls are feasible; however, rubber dam isolation is ideal.

Caries removal

Local anesthesia before caries removal is necessary if the cavity is deep. According to the minimally invasive principle, select the burs according to the size of the cavity. No need to do extra extension or anatomic wear, just completely removal of caries. A laser system approved for hard tissue can be used to gain access to the depth of the lesion and to complete caries removal. The preparation, which should not extend to the occlusal contact marks, is washed, dried, and examined [Figure 5 - 2 (C) and (D)].

Etching

Use a brush, small sponge, cotton pellet or applicator provided by the manufacturer to place 35% phosphate acid widely across the enamel surface to be sealed for 20 seconds. For primary teeth, extend the etching to 40 - 60 s is necessary. Some advocate preparing the enamel for sealant application with an aluminum oxide air abrasion system or a laser system approved for hard-tissue procedures. To date, studies indicate that additional acid-etching is needed after each of these techniques to allow for adequate resin bonding to the enamel [Figure 5 - 2 (E) and (F)].

Rinsing and dry

The tooth is thoroughly rinsed for approximately 30 - 40 s and completely dried with a compressed air stream that is free of oil contaminants until the etched enamel exhibiting characteristic frosty appearance [Figure 5 -2 (G)].

Place the bonding agents

- A thin layer of bonding agent is applied to the cavity. A stream of air must be used to thin the bonding agent and to prevent pooling of bonding agent in the cavity. The materials are polymerized with curing light following the manufacturer's instructions.
- Although it is recommended to avoid moisture contamination whenever possible during sealant application, the use of a dentin-bonding agent as part of the technique appears to be warranted. Furthermore, the use of a dentin-bonding agent is recommended in clinical situations that do not lend themselves to strict isolation—for example, when newly erupted teeth are sealed or when patient cooperation is not ideal.
- The use of a dentin-bonding agent is also advantageous on the buccal surfaces of molars, which traditionally have shown a lower retention rate than the occlusal surfaces of teeth. When used, the bonding agent must be thoroughly air-dried across the surface to be sealed to avoid a thick layer of adhesive residue [Figure 5 -2 (H) and (I)].

Fill the cavity

The flowable or condensable resin was used to restore the anatomic form of the teeth, avoiding the incorporation of air bubbles. The resin was then polymerized with curing light [Figure 5 -2 (J)].

Application of light-cured sealant

- A light-curing sealant is placed over the remaining susceptible areas and brushed into the pits and fissures. Polymerized with curing light [Figure 5 -2 (K) and (L)].
- The use of flowable composite systems is also gaining in popularity because they are easy to apply and evidence shows that less microleakage occurs with these systems than when teeth are restored with condensable composite resins, such as sealant materials that have slightly more filler than filled sealants. Therefore, the practical results of sealing with a flowable or a filled sealant should be the same.

Occlusal check

Remove the isolation and use articulating paper to check for occlusal interferences. All centric stops should be on the enamel. A small-particle diamond bur with a high-speed handpiece can be used to remove excess restorative material and ensure centric stops on the enamel [Figure 5 -2 (M) and (N)].

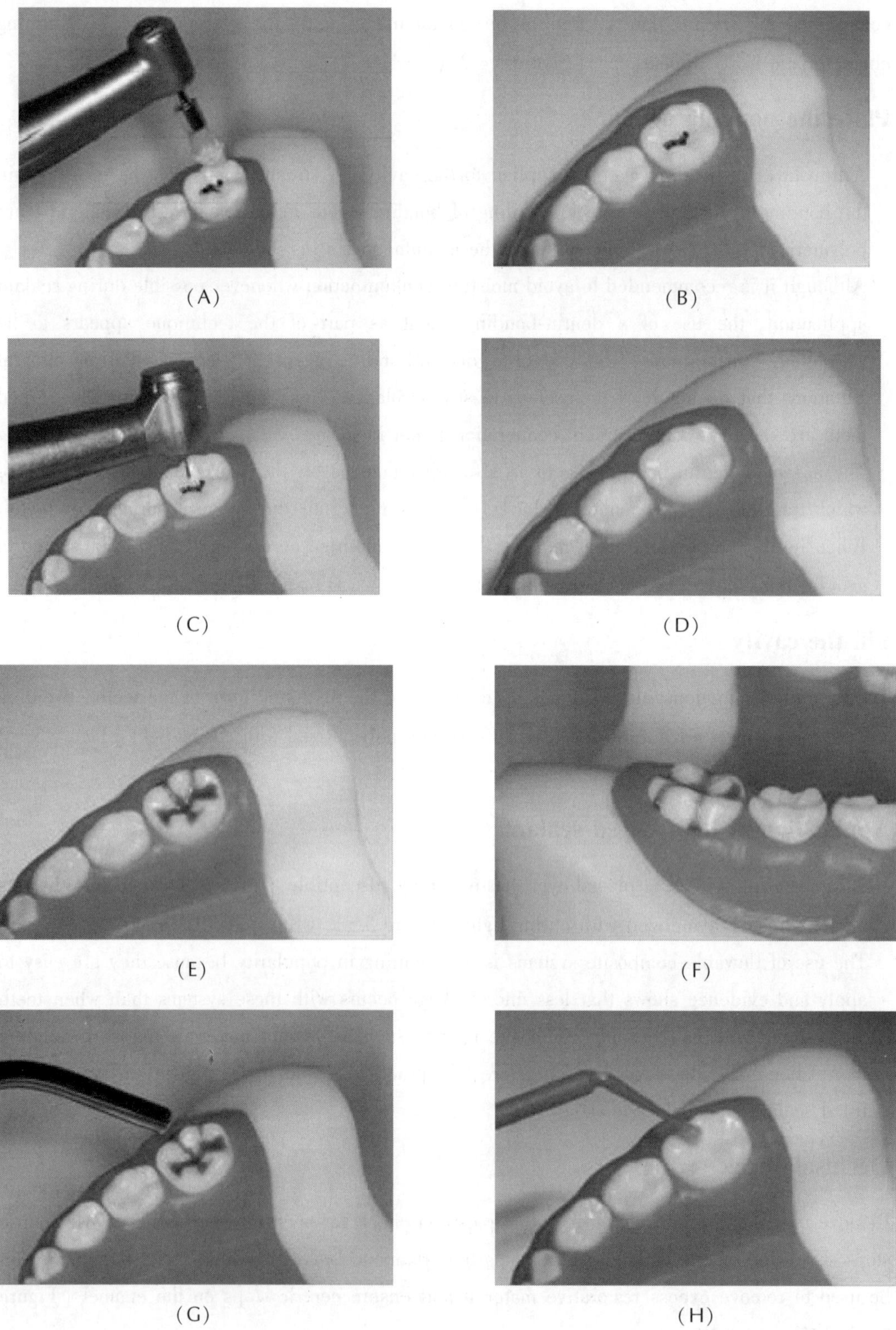

(A) (B)

(C) (D)

(E) (F)

(G) (H)

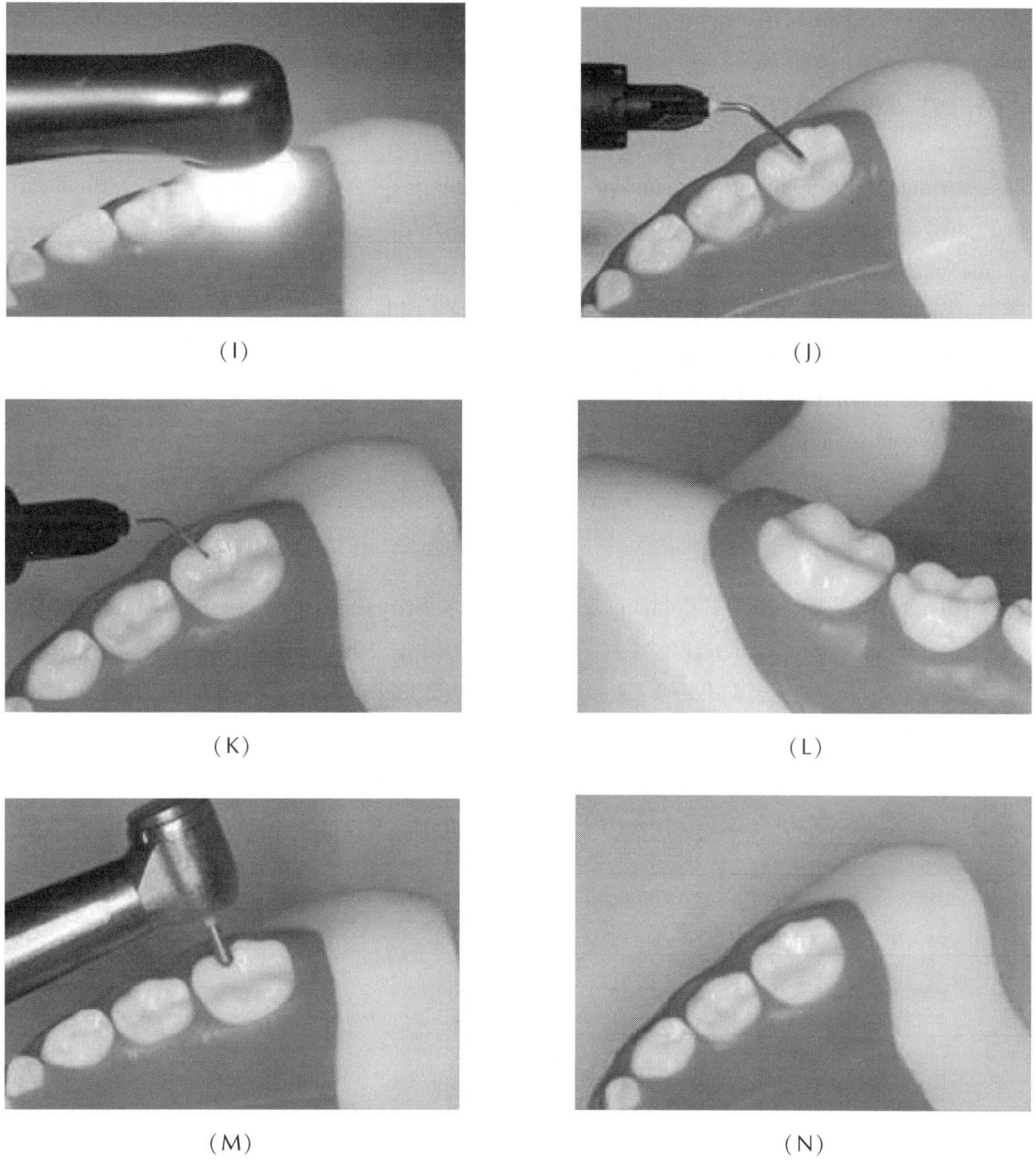

(I) (J) (K) (L) (M) (N)

Figure 5 - 2 Procedures of PRR.

Tips

1. If the bottom of the cavity is at the medium or deep 1/3 of dentin, indirect capping with $Ca(OH)_2$ agent and resin filling of the cavity should be done before etching.
2. Gently place the etching agent on the enamel surface avoiding breaking the enamel rods. The lingual grooves of maxillary molars and the buccal grooves of mandibular molars are also commonly etched.
3. Avoiding the incorporation of air bubbles when brushing the sealant into the groves. Remove

the extra sealant before light curing, especially those around the free gingiva.

Process assessment for students' practice

The instructor will grade the students' practice according to:

- Proper site and amount of caries removal. No need to do extra extension or anatomic wear, just completely removal of the caries;
- The etching agent was widely placed on all the susceptible grooves and fissures;
- No air bubbles or extra sealant when placing the sealant;
- The resin restoration and sealant are properly done;
- Ensure centric stops when checking the occlusion.

References

[1] Houpt M, Fuks A, Eidelman E. The preventive resin (composite resin/sealant) restoration: nine-year results [J]. Quintessence Int. 1994, 25 (3): 155 - 159.

[2] Dean JA, Jones JE, Walker Vinson LA. McDonald and Avery's dentistry for the child and adolescent [M]. 10th ed. St. Louis: Elsevier, 2016.

CHAPTER 6

RESIN FILLED STRIP CROWN RESTORATION FOR PRIMARY INCISORS

Introduction to strip crown restoration technique

Large-sized restoration in primary incisor is a difficult challenge to the dentist. An alternative restoration for the severely damaged anterior tooth is the resin filled crown form. Strip crown is a prefabricated, transparent strip crown for primary anterior tooth applications. The strip crown is ideal for utilization with chemical or light-cured composites, which is automatically contoured restorative material to match natural dentition.

The clinical indications for strip crown restoration

1. Restoration for primary incisors with extensive and/or multiple caries lesions.
2. Restoration for primary incisors with Class Ⅳ cavity.
3. Restorations for hypoplastic primary teeth that cannot be adequately restored with bonded restorations.
4. Restorations for teeth with hereditary anomalies, such as dentinogenesis imperfecta or amelogenesis imperfecta.
5. Restorations for pulptomized or pulpectomized primary teeth when there is an increased danger of fracture of the remaining coronal tooth structure.
6. Restorations for fractured teeth if the teeth could be saved.

The advantages of strip crown restoration

1. Strip crown is beautiful and lifelike, and can restore the anatomical form and adjacent relationship better than traditional bonded restoration.
2. Strip crown is very convenient to recover the outline and contour of the anterior teeth and will shorten the operation time.
3. Compared with direct resin filling, the shedding rate decreases significantly.

The life span of the strip crown due to several factors

1. Susceptibility to the technique of the operator.
2. The cooperation of patient during the treatment.
3. If the patient is to bite things with or without the anterior teeth.
4. Individual oral conditions.
5. Oral hygiene.

These aspects should be explained to both parent and patient, as well as home care instructions. The replacement may be occasionally necessary, depending on the length of time the tooth will remain in the mouth.

The objective of lab practice

1. To master the procedures of tooth preparation and strip crown restoration.
2. To be familiar with the indications and contradiction for strip crowns applied.
3. To know the advantages and the factors affect the life span of strip crowns.

Materials and instruments

1. Training model with plastic primary incisor.
2. For tooth preparation: high-speed handpiece, low-speed handpiece [Figure 6 - 1 (A) and (B)].
3. Burs: diamond bur, very thin flamed-shaped diamond bur or conical diamond, wheel-shaped diamond bur [Figure 6 - 1 (A) and (B)].
4. Curved-tip scissor [Figure 6 - 1 (C)].
5. 37% phosphoric acid solution, flowable composite resin, bonding agents, visible light-cured sealant, visible curing light [Figure 6 - 1 (D)].
6. Strip crown [Figure 6 - 1 (E) and (F)].

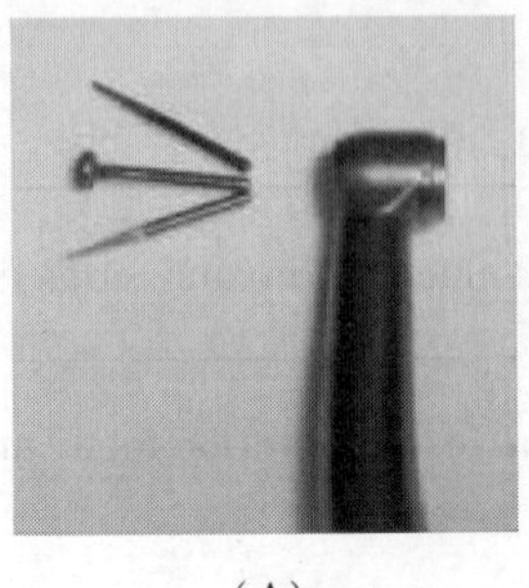
(A)

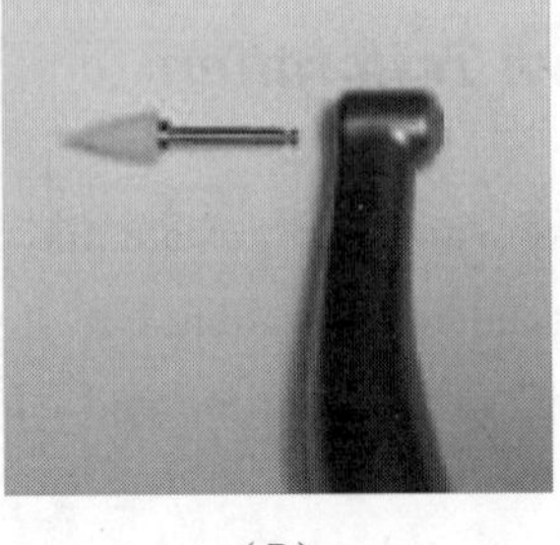
(B)

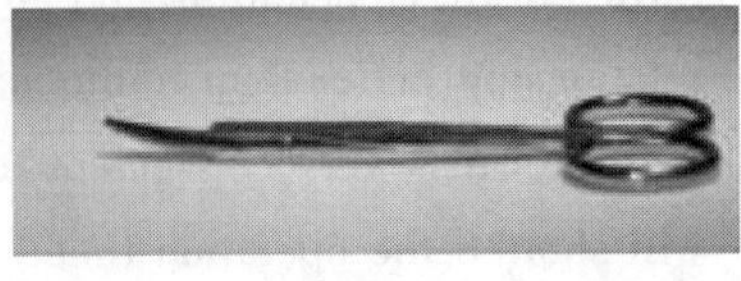
(C)

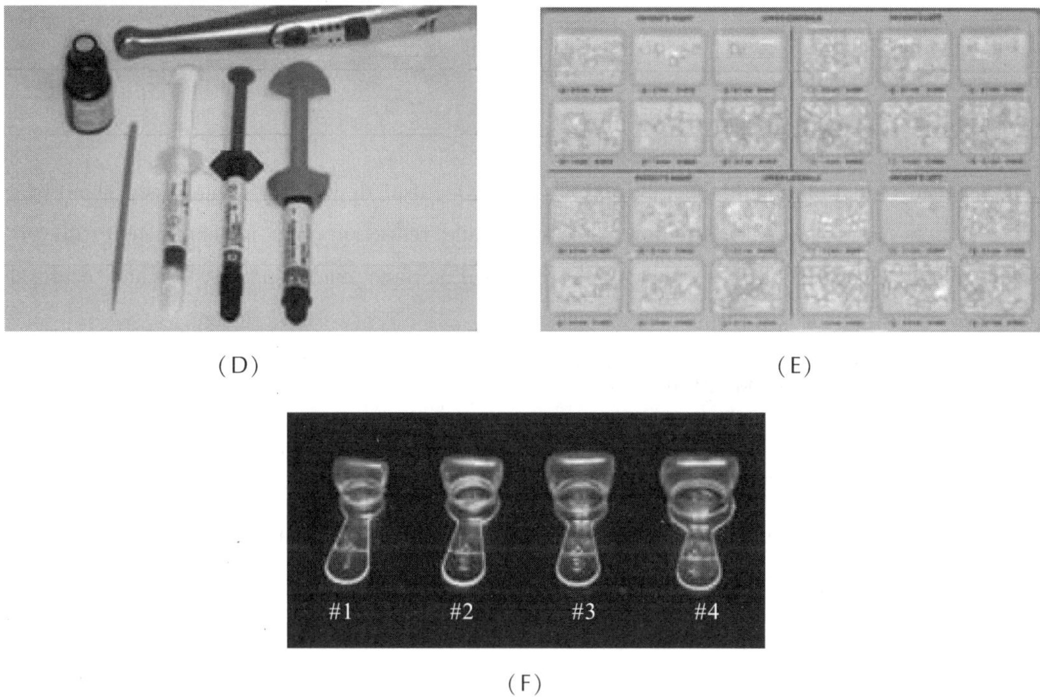

(D) (E)

(F)

Figure 6 −1 Materials and instruments.

Preparation of teeth (*optional*)

1. Anesthetize the appropriate area if needed.
2. Place the rubber dam. Much of the preparation can be accomplished under the rubber dam.
3. All carious tooth structure should be removed before preparing the tooth for a crown. Use a round bur to uncover the carious lesion for complete visualization. Using the slow speed handpiece, the largest round bur appropriate to the size of the lesion should be used to remove the carious dentin.
4. Place a calcium hydroxide base in areas where caries removal was deep and near the pulp, and fill the cavity with resin.

Practice steps

Strip crown selection

A variety of clear plastic crown form sizes are available and one should be selected that most closely complements the remaining dentition or final preparation. The contra-lateral tooth may be used as a guide for this selection [Figure 6 −2 (A)].

Tooth preparation

• Occlusal preparation

The occlusal reduction should be uniformly 1 mm. Occlusal depth-cuts 1 mm deep should be used to help assure proper reduction. The remaining reduction may be completed with the wheel-shaped diamond bur as long as the reduced surface maintains the original occlusal contours [Figure 6 - 2 (B) and (C)].

• Mesial and distal preparation

Mesial and distal reductions are made with the bur (very thin flamed-shaped diamond bur) positioned parallel to the long axis of the tooth. Be very careful not to damage the proximal surface of the adjacent tooth. The mesial and distal walls should converge slightly with gingival margins ending in feather edges without any ledges [Figure 6 - 2 (D)].

• Lingual and facial preparation

Lingual reduction should be uniformly 0.5 mm and the facial reduction should be uniformly 1 mm, the four axial line angles are rounded to maintain the general contour of the surfaces of the crown [Figure 6 - 2 (E) to (F)].

All margins of the crown must be smooth and end in a feather edge by using thin flamed-shaped diamond bur or conical diamond [Figure 6 - 2 (G)]. If sufficient tooth structure remains, this feather margin should be supragingival. Leave as much enamel as possible to aid in retention by means of acid etching. After the preparation a strip crown is selected.

• Strip crown trimming

Using small curved-tip scissors, the crown form should be trimmed to fit the preparation. Once the crown form is properly trimmed and trial fitted, one or two small vent holes should be placed on the lingual at the mesial and/or distal incisal edges to minimize air bubbles in the resin [Figure 6 - 2 (H) to (J)]. Any remaining unprepared enamel should be roughened slightly with a diamond bur.

• Tooth etching

The entire preparation should be etched with 30% - 50% phosphoric acid for one minute on primary teeth. The preparation should be washed with water and dried thoroughly without any contamination by saliva [Figure 6 - 2 (K)].

• Bonding restoration

A universal bonding agent is applied to the entire preparation according to the manufacturer's instructions. The crown should be appropriately filled with the proper shade of the resin with a composite applicator. The filled crown form is fitted over the preparation to its proper position and the excess resin removed at the cervical margin with an explorer. The resin is light-cured and polymerized for 30 seconds each on the lingual, facial and incisal surfaces according to the manufacturer's instructions [Figure 6-2 (L) to (S)].

- **Polish and finish**

The crown form is carefully split away from the cured resin by cutting down the lingual (preferably) or labial of the crown with a bur until it can be peeled off with an explorer [Figure 6-2 (T)]. The margins are finished down with a flame-shaped diamond bur. Any necessary adjustments for incisal length, occlusion, or anatomy can be accomplished with sandpaper discs or finishing burs. The best finish is that imparted by the crown form. Do as little finishing as possible. If the restoration needs any final smoothing, finishing strips or prophy paste with a rubber cup may be used. Be sure to check for any occlusal disharmonies [Figure 6-2 (U) and (V)].

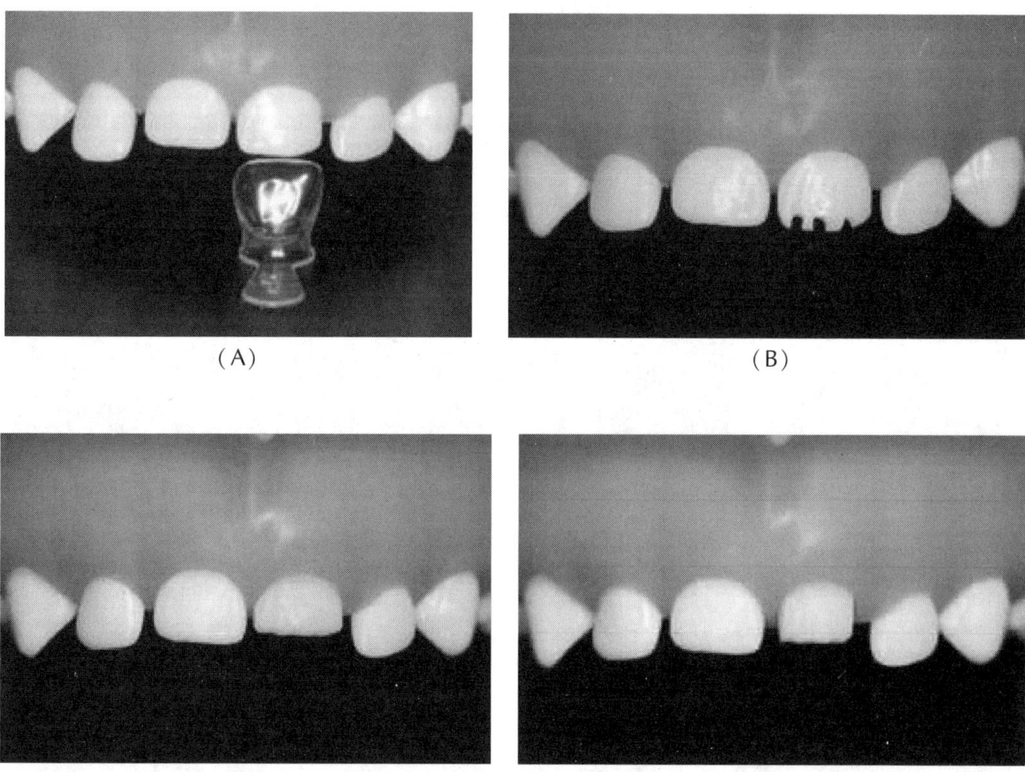

(A) (B)

(C) (D)

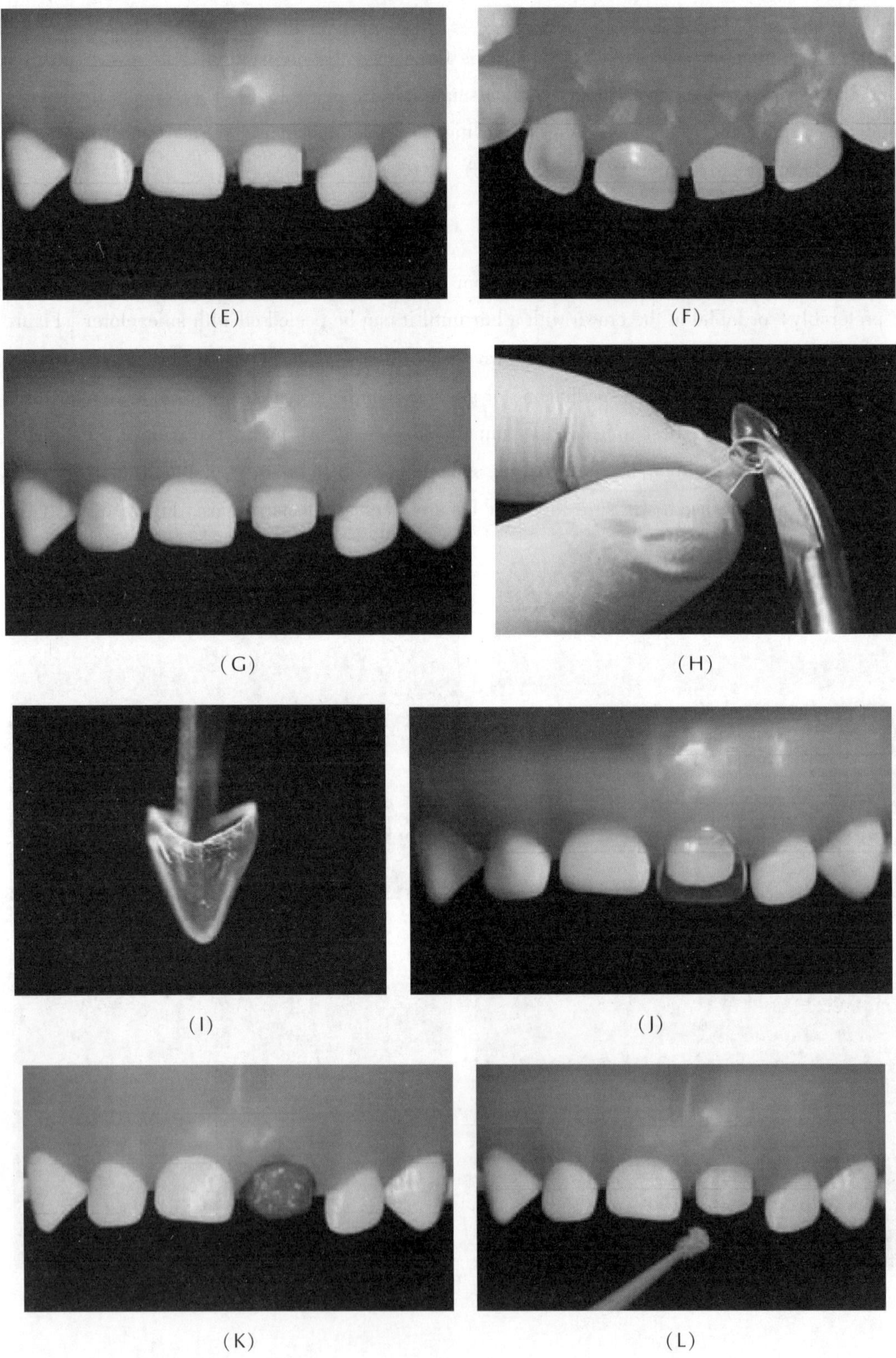

(E) (F) (G) (H) (I) (J) (K) (L)

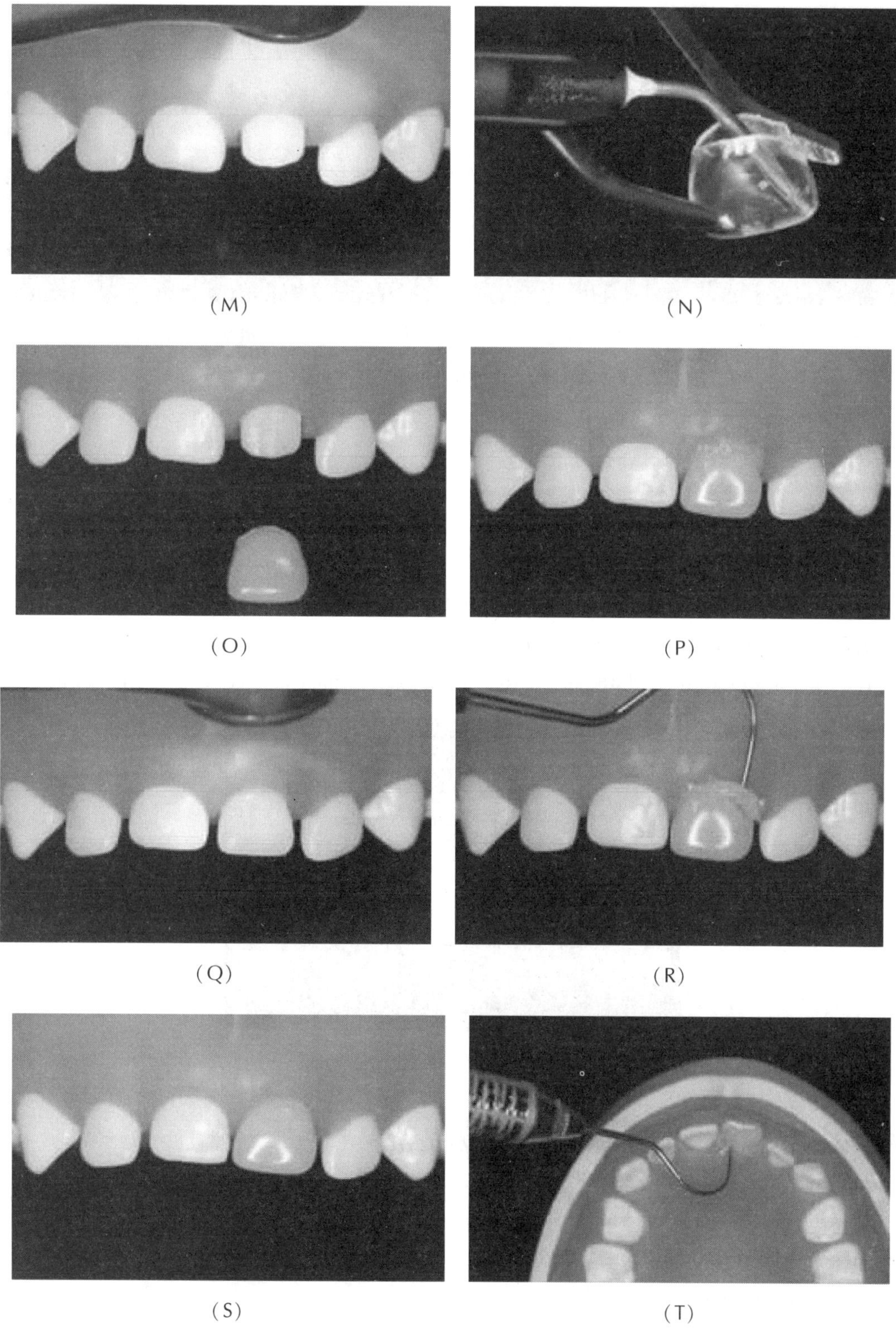

(M) (N)

(O) (P)

(Q) (R)

(S) (T)

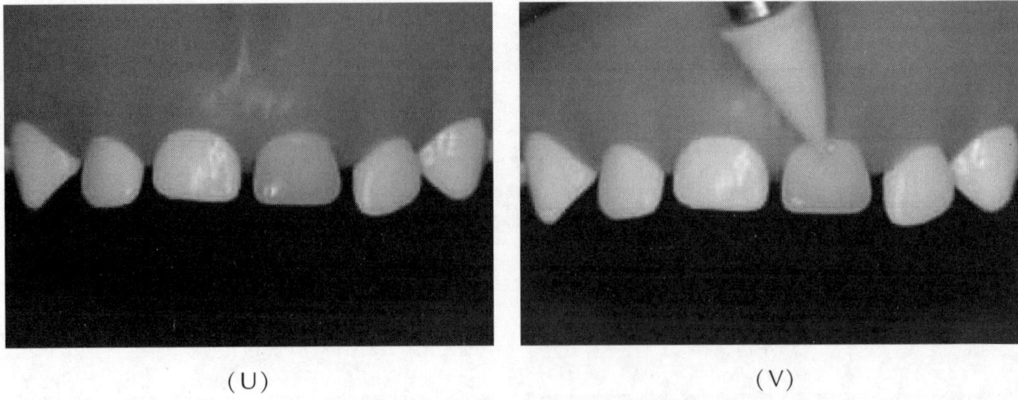

(U) (V)

Figure 6 -2 Tooth preparations steps.

Tips

1. When preparing the proximal surfaces, care must be taken not to damage the adjacent tooth surface.
2. It is also helpful to vent the incisal edge of the crown with an explorer to both prevent inner air bubbles and lead the flow of resin (Figure 6 -3).
3. Hold the strip crown carefully and if you fell the crown then it is hard to find it again.

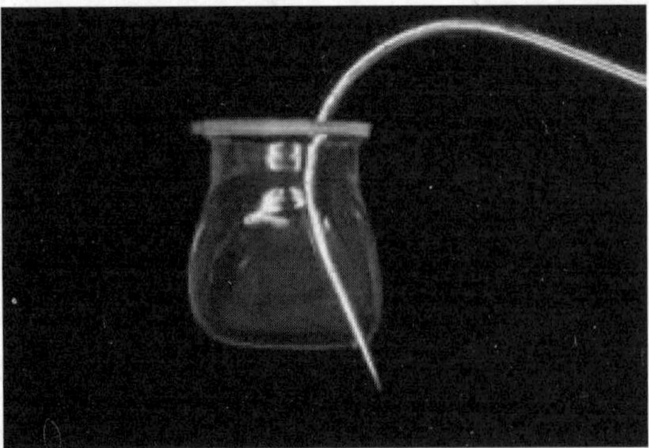

Figure 6 -3 Vent hole for strip crown.

Process assessment for students' practice

The instructor will grade the students' practice according to:

- Proper tooth preparation for all surfaces;
- Careful protection for proximal teeth;
- Proper trimming for the crown;
- Proper fitting of the crown;
- Neat final adhesion and proper occlusion.

References

Waggoner WF. Restoring primary anterior teeth: updated for 2014 [J]. Pediatr Dent, 2015, 37 (2): 163 - 170.

CHAPTER 7
STAINLESS STEEL CROWN RESTORATION FOR PRIMARY MOLARS

Introduction to stainless steel crown restoration technique

Stainless steel crown (SSC), also known as "preformed metal crown", was introduced by Humphrey in 1950 and is now most frequently used in caries restorations for primary molars. In addition, SSCs can also be applied to young permanent molars as an interim restoration procedure, they would be further replaced with permanent restoration until late adolescence or early adulthood.

SSC has shown significant clinical success and is considered a favorable restoration for multiple-surface and large carious lesions. The SSCs are pre-trimmed, belled and crimped for fast and easy placement. Therefore, the restoration is relatively convenient comparing to traditional crown restoration. The morphology of SSCs accurately mimics the anatomy of primary or young permanent molars and offers a comfortable fit for pediatric patients. Furthermore, the superior durability with low replacement rate is also a major advantage of SSC. The clinical failure rate of SSC restoration is about four times lower than that of amalgam restoration for Class II cavities.

SSC restoration is not recommended for children allergic to stainless steel material, neither for teeth approaching exfoliation or replaced by a succeeding permanent tooth.

The removal of placed SSCs may be suggested when symptoms and signs of allergy to the SSC were noticed, or other situations that SSC could not be kept in mouth.

The clinical indications for SSC

1. Restoration for primary or young permanent molars with extensive and/or multiple-surface caries lesions.
2. Restorations for hypoplastic primary or young permanent molars that cannot be adequately restored with bonded restorations.
3. Restorations for teeth with hereditary anomalies, such as dentinogenesis imperfecta or amelogenesis imperfecta.

4. Restorations for pulptomized or pulpectomized primary or young permanent molars when there is an increased danger of fracture of the remaining coronal tooth structure.
5. Restorations for fractured teeth after necessary treatment.
6. Restorations for primary teeth to be used as abutments for appliances.
7. Attachments for habit-breaking and orthodontic appliances.

The objective of lab practice

1. To master the indications and contradictions for SSC restoration.
2. To be familiar with the procedures of tooth preparation and SSC restoration.
3. To know the circumstances of SSC removal.

Materials and instruments

1. Training model with plastic right mandibular second primary molar (#85) and opposing model [Figure 7-1 (A)].
2. Stainless steel crown (in a set with 6 different sizes) [Figure 7-1 (B)].
3. High-speed handpiece for tooth preparation [Figure 7-1 (C)].
4. Low-speed handpiece for crown polishing after trimming [Figure 7-1 (C)].
5. Burs: thin flame-shaped diamond bur, wheel-shaped diamond bur, rubber polishing stone [Figure 7-1 (C)].
6. Crown-crimping pliers, Crown-contouring pliers, Curved-beak pliers [Figure 7-1 (D)].
7. Curved-tip scissor [Figure 7-1 (E)].
8. Glass ionomer cement for crown luting [Figure 7-1 (F) and (G)].

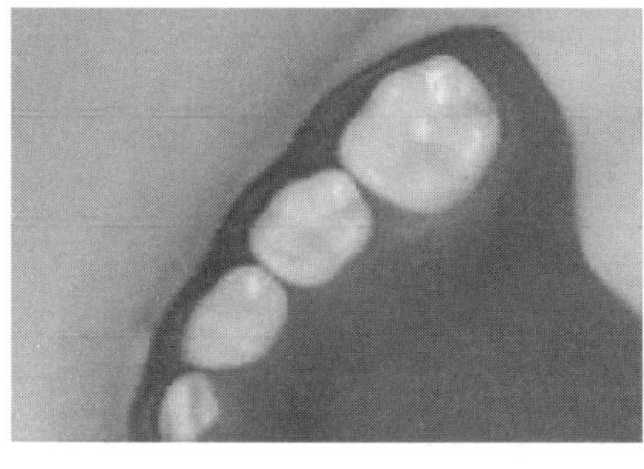

(A)

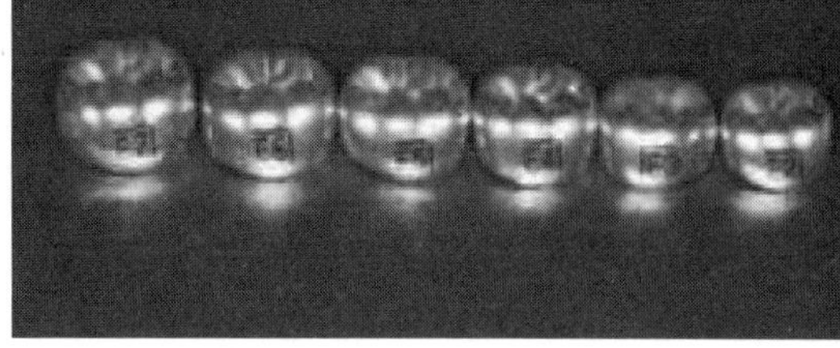

(B)

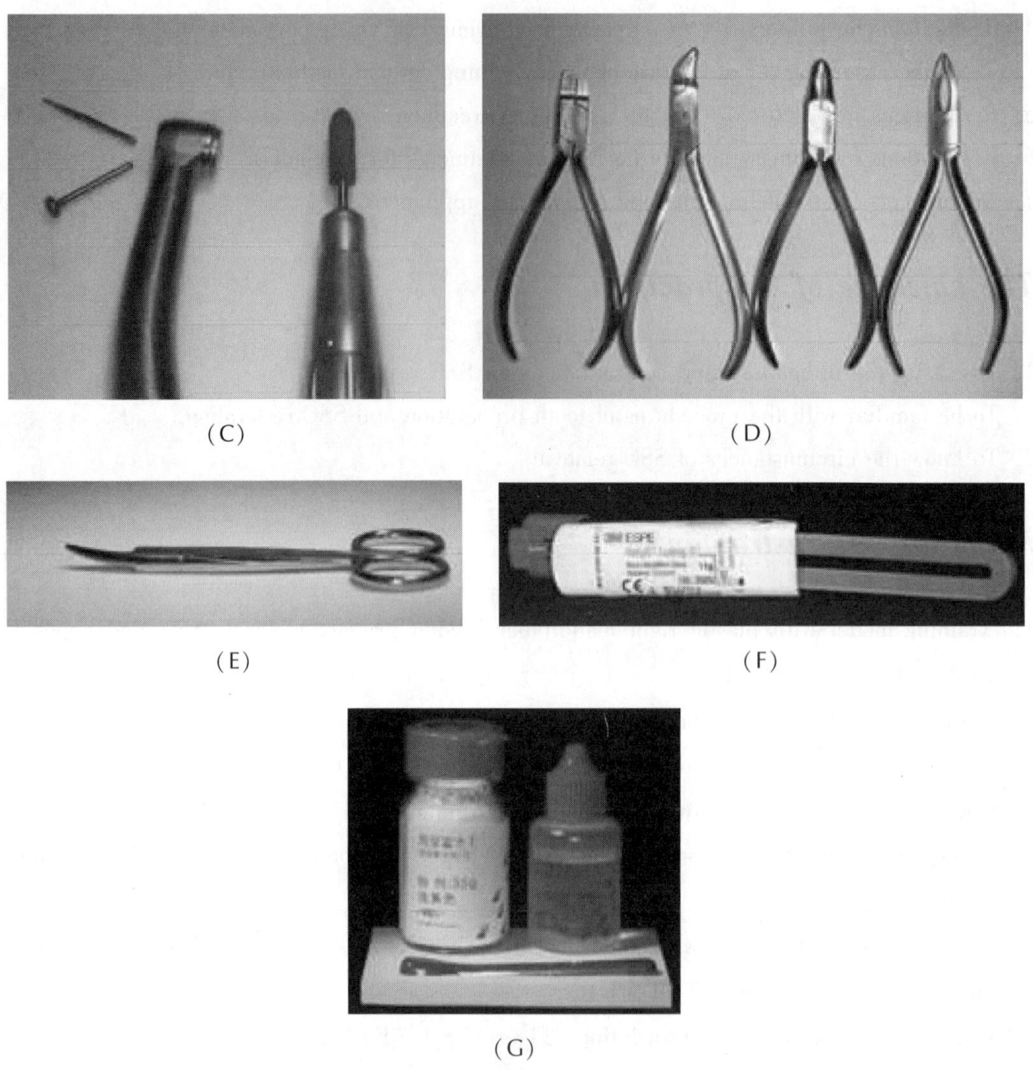

(C) (D)

(E) (F)

(G)

Figure 7 −1 Materials and instruments.

Practice steps

Tooth preparation

- The occlusal reduction should be uniformly 1 −1. 5 mm. Reduce the contour of the occlusal surface and the cusps of the tooth by using wheel-shaped diamond bur at high speed [Figure 7 −2 (A) to (C)].
- Mesial and distal reductions are made and the proximal contact with adjacent teeth was broken by a very thin flamed-shaped diamond bur at high speed. The bur should be positioned parallel to the long axis of the tooth. Be very careful and not to damage the proximal surface of the adjacent teeth. The mesial and distal walls should converge slightly

with gingival margins ending in feather edges without any ledges. The proximal surfaces are reduced for approximately 0.5 mm [Figure 7-2 (D) and (E)].

- Remove all sharp line and point angles by using thin flamed-shaped diamond bur at high speed. The four axial line angles are rounded to maintain the general contour of the surfaces of the crown. All cervical margins of the crown must be smooth and end in a feather edge [Figure 7-2 (F)]. Not necessary to reduce the buccal or lingual surfaces in lab practice.

Crown selection

Determine the diameter of the space between the two adjacent teeth to the prepared tooth. Caliper can be used to aid the distance determination for beginners. Select the smallest crown that could completely cover the preparation and gain a proper fit [Figure 7-2 (G)].

Crown trimming and try-in

Adjust the shape and margin of SSC by using crown-crimping plier and curved-tip scissors. Usually, the crowns are pre-contoured and pre-crimpled, but further contouring and crimping may be required to close any open margins to improve the fitting. The crown-crimping plier usually is used at the cervical third of the crown and produces a beveled gingival margin. The crown should be adapted so that it will "snap-on" securely into place. Gross trimming of excess crown material can be accomplished with curved-tip scissors. [Figure 7-2 (H) to (M)].

Polish

Use a rubber polishing stone at low speed to polish the crown and remove sharp edges when necessary.

Occlusion check and cement

Prior to cementation, check the occlusion to opposing teeth and the subgingival extension of the crown margins. Use glass ionomer cement to cement the SSC to the tooth [Figure 7-2 (N) to (O)].

Clean and finish

Clean excess cement around margins and interproximal space. Excess glass ionomer cement can be rinsed away easily before it sets. Check for proper final seating of SSC and the occlusion [Figure 7-2 (P) and (Q)].

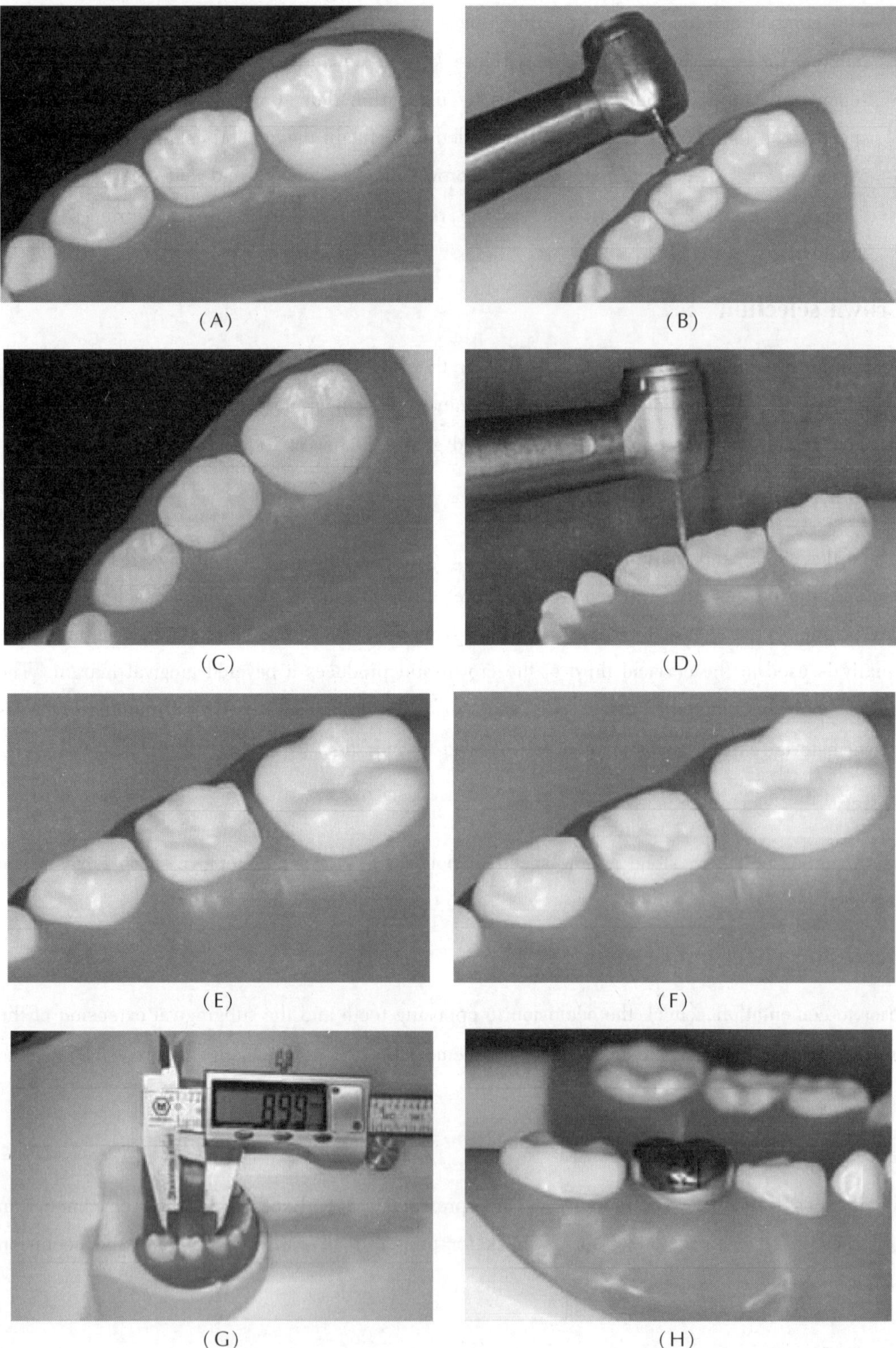

(A) (B)

(C) (D)

(E) (F)

(G) (H)

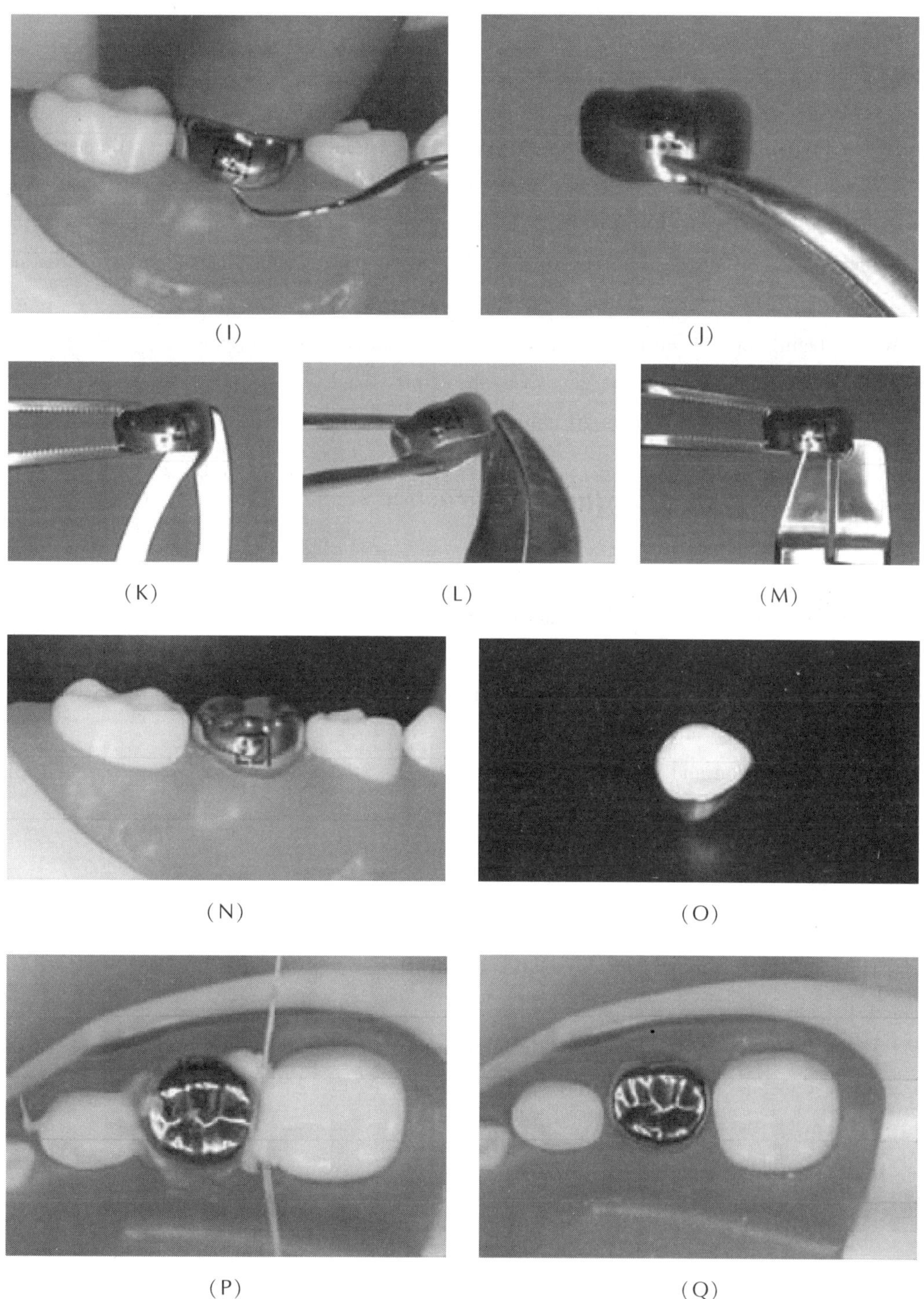

(I) (J) (K) (L) (M) (N) (O) (P) (Q)

Figure 7 −2 Tooth preparations.

Tips

1. When preparing the proximal surfaces, care must be taken not to damage adjacent tooth surfaces in the clinic. Wooden wedge or rubber band can be applied to the proximal space before the preparation and provide slight separation.
2. Usually, there is no need to prepare the buccal/lingual/palatal surface unless a distinct bulge is present and SSC cannot be placed.
3. When placing the SSC on the tooth, make sure the gingival margin extending 0.5 – 1.0 mm beneath the free margin of the gingiva in the clinic.
4. A piece of floss with two knots 20 mm apart facilitates cleaning the interproximal space.

Process assessment for students' practice

The instructor will grade the students' practice according to:

- Proper tooth preparation for all surfaces.
- Careful protection for proximal teeth.
- Proper trimming and polishing for the crown.
- Proper fitting of the crown.
- Neat final adhesion and proper occlusion.

References

[1] Randall RC, Vrijhoef MM, Wilson NH, et al. Efficacy of preformed metal crowns vs. amalgam restorations in primary molars: a systematic review [J]. J Am Dent Assoc, 2000, 131 (3): 337 – 343.

[2] Zheng LW, Zou J, Xia B, et al. Restoration of preformed metal crown on dental caries of primary molars [J]. Inter J Stomatol, 2017, 44 (2): 125 – 129.

CHAPTER 8

MANUFACTURE OF SPACE MAINTENANCE FOR EARLY LOSS OF PRIMARY MOLARS

Introduction to space maintenance

When primary teeth are lost as a result of caries, ectopic eruption or trauma, the occlusion must be assessed carefully to determine if space maintenance is necessary. Early loss of deciduous teeth can result in the loss of arch length leading to malocclusion. The maintenance of arch length in the primary, mixed and early permanent dentition is important for the normal development of the occlusion. Space maintenance can often prevent space loss, either prevent the development of a later malocclusion or reduce its severity. It was observed that early loss of upper second deciduous molars modifies greater the vertical axis of the permanent molars than the premature loss of first upper primary molar. First upper deciduous molar loss causes an acceleration eruption of first premolar, which will produce a distal inclination of both permanent molars. The use of space maintainers after premature loss of the second upper primary molar is the last solution in preventing tridimensional lesions in the dental arch and occlusion.

Whether to engage in space maintenance and which technique to use must be based on a careful assessment of the total patient and their clinical status. Generally, space maintenance is appropriate when Class I skeletal and dental relationships are present, when adequate space (as determined by a space analysis) is available, and when the facial profile is well balanced with appropriate lip posture. Even in the presence of these qualifications, poor patient cooperation, certain medical conditions and/or poor oral hygiene may ultimately contraindicate space maintenance. The indications for selecting a specific appliance must be based on numerous factors such as which teeth (or tooth) are (or is) missing, which teeth (or tooth) are (or is) available for abutments, should fixed or removable appliances be used, and what is the position and stage of development of the unerupted teeth.

Space maintainers can be fixed or removable. The types of space maintainers include semi-fixed space maintainers (consisting of distal guide plate space maintainers, full crown or band and loop space maintainers, filling space maintainers), fixed space maintainers (consisting of tongue bow space maintainers, Nance bow space maintainers) and removable space maintainers. Band and loop space maintainers have fewer problems than other types.

The indications for the use and loop space maintainers include the following:

· Early loss of first deciduous molar.
· A case of early loss of the second deciduous molar after the eruption of the first permanent molar.
· Early loss of bilateral deciduous molars and difficulty in using other space maintainers.

The objective of lab practice

1. To master the indications, function and the types of space maintainers.
2. To be familiar to the manufacture procedures.

Materials and instruments

1. Mixed dentition mandibular training model with the early loss of the second deciduous molar.
2. Stainless steel band kit [Figure 8 - 1 (A) and (B)].
3. Curved-tip scissor [Figure 8 - 1 (C)].
4. Stainless steel wire in 0.9 - 1.0mm diameter [Figure 8 - 1 (D)].
5. Excising forceps [Figure 8 - 1 (D)].
6. Marking pen.
7. Clasp forceps [Figure 8 - 1 (E)].
8. Band pusher [Figure 8 - 1 (E)].

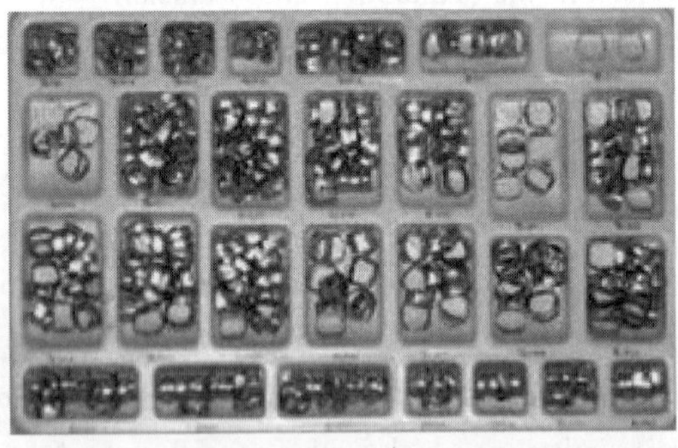

(A)

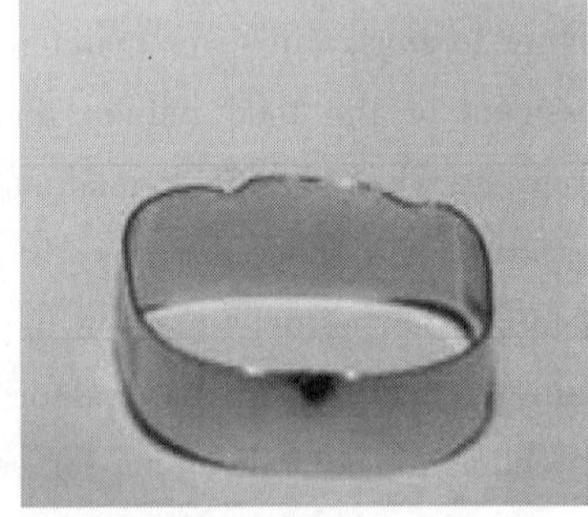

(B)

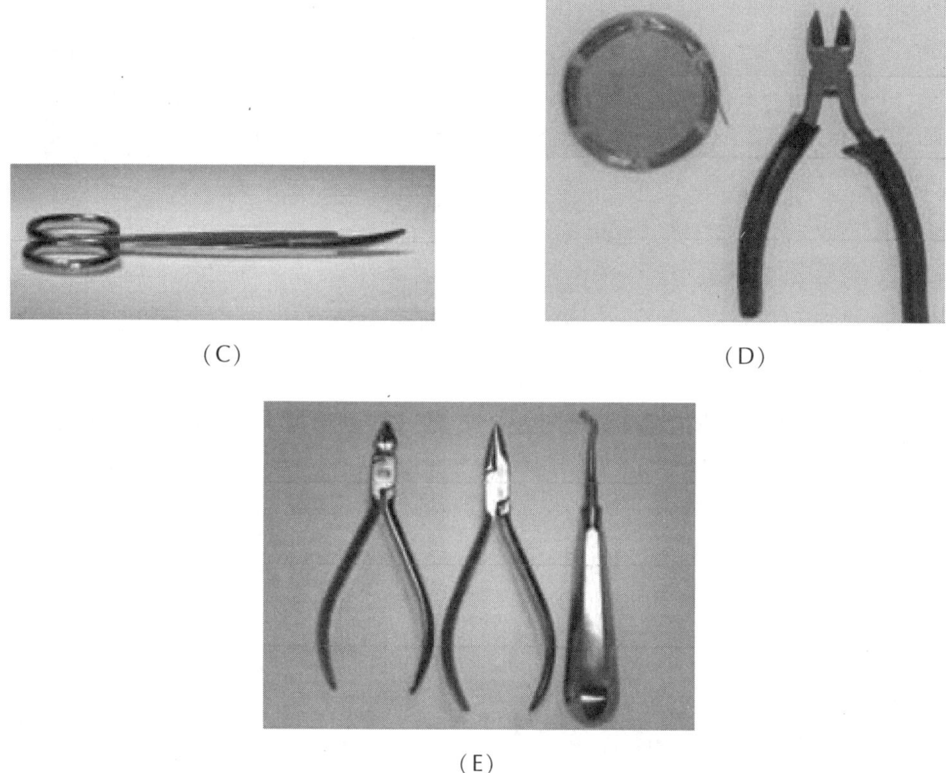

(C) (D)

(E)

Figure 8 - 1 Materials and instruments.

Practice steps

Band fitting

1. Fit a preformed stainless steel orthodontic band to the adjacent first permanent tooth chosen for an abutment [Figure 8 - 2 (A) and (B)]. Cut off the occlusal surface and gingival redundant edges, so that the band rings work in the corresponding parts of the abutment teeth [Figure 8 - 2 (C)]. The occlusion should not be obstructed clinically.
2. Assuming the fit is good, with no voids around the circumference, the band can be contoured into the anatomical grooves of the tooth. This can be accomplished with careful lateral pressure using a band pusher [Figure 8 - 2 (D)], on the facial, lingual, mesial, and distal occlusal margins of the band. Use proper finger rest and guard against the band pusher slipping.
3. The banded tooth are checked for the final contour and fit. Have an instructor check the fitted bands.

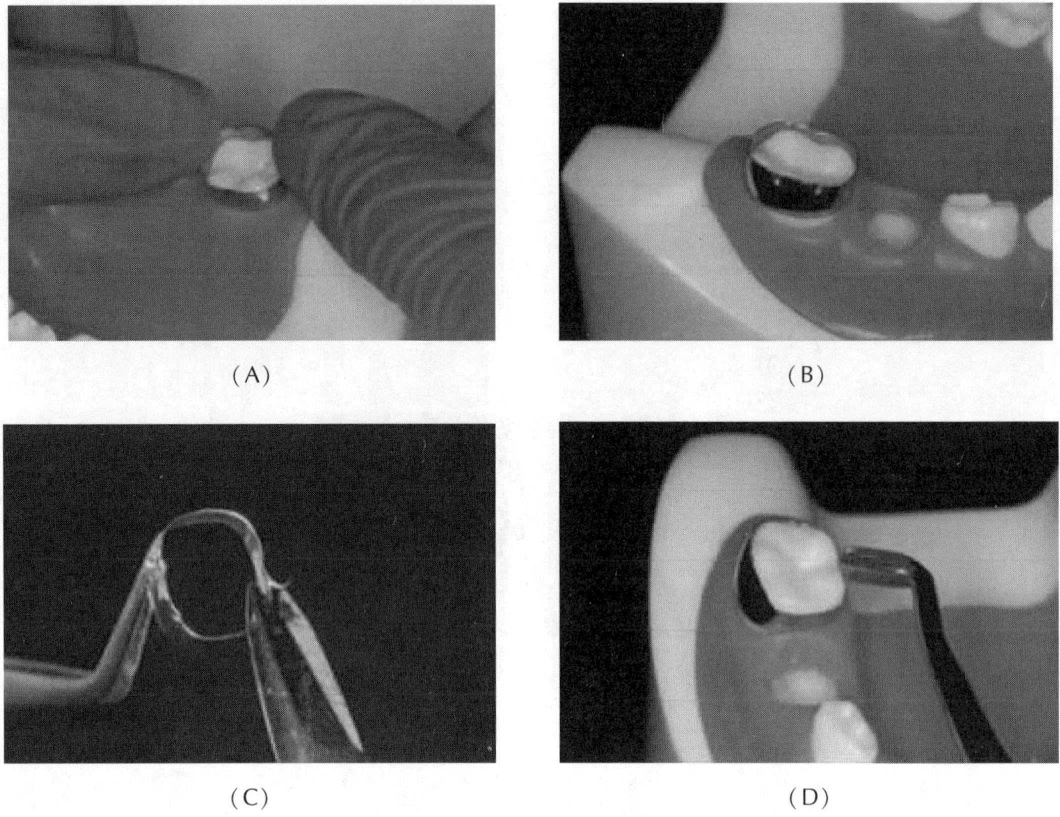

(A) (B) (C) (D)

Figure 8 - 2 Band fitting.

Loop making

1. Bend an 0. 9 mm diameter stainless steel wire into a loop to contact the distal surface of the first deciduous molar at the height of contour [Figure 8 - 3 (A) and (B)].
2. First, the stainless steel wire is bent into "U" shape, and the end is identical with the distal surface of the first deciduous molar [Figure 8 - 3 (C) to (F)]. The buccolingual width of "U" shape is slightly larger than that between the buccal and lingual axial angles of the first deciduous molar and the first permanent molar.
3. The end of the wire should reach distal 1/3 of the crown of the first permanent molar, and its height should reach middle 1/3 of the clinical crown [Figure 8 - 3 (G) to (J)]. The wire is kept 1. 5 mm off the soft tissue [Figure 8 - 3 (K)].

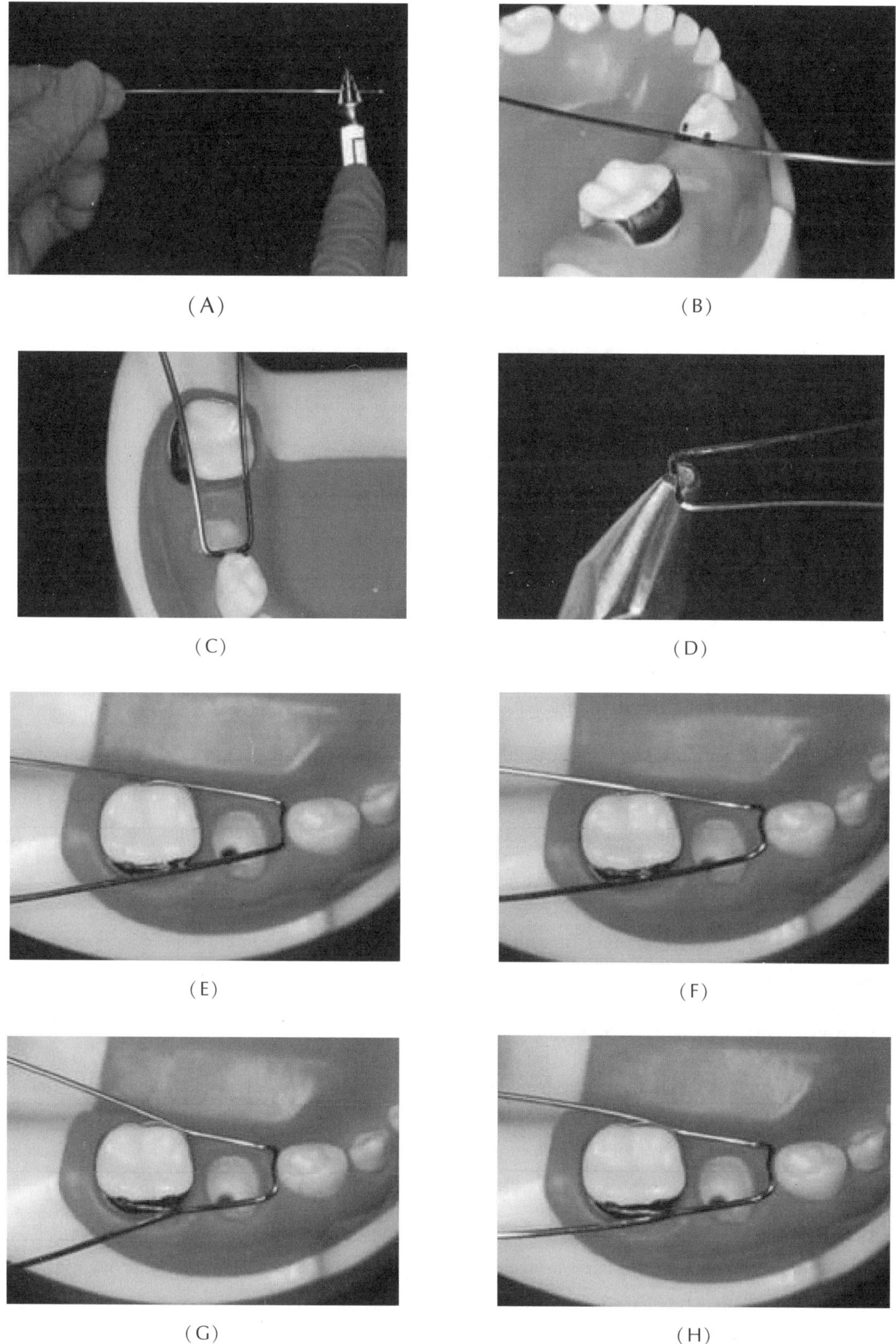

(A) (B) (C) (D) (E) (F) (G) (H)

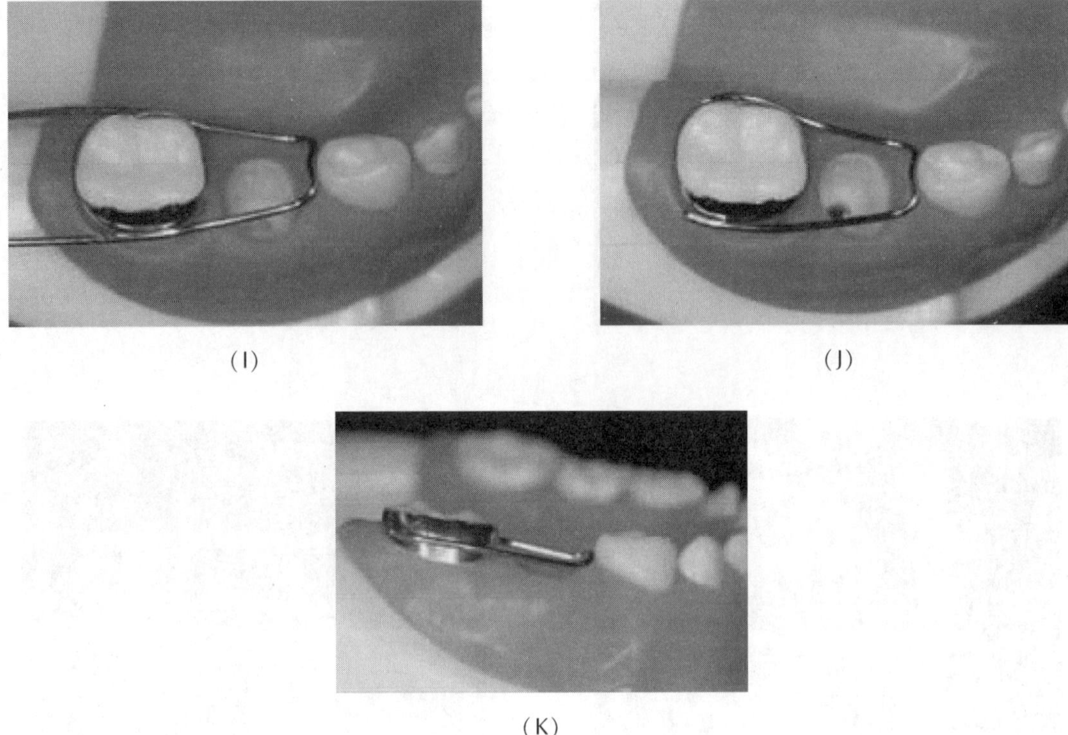

(I) (J)

(K)

Figure 8 - 3 Loop making process.

Welding (optional practice)

The free end of the bent loop is fixed with wax and gypsum, then the welding part is coated with welding enzymes, welding gold is placed. The welding part and the welding gold are heated by the external flame of the welding gun so that the welding gold completely wraps the steel wire.

Polishing (optional practice)

Remove the welded wire retainer from the model without distortion, remove the excess welding gold with a drill, and finally polish it.

Cementation (optional practice)

Band and loop space maintainer are bonded to abutments with glass ionomer cementing powder.

Tips

1. Band and loop space maintainers should not interfere with occlusion.
2. Polishing the edge of the band to avoid the formation of ulcers by irritating oral mucosa.
3. Attention should be paid to preventing the slippage of the band ring from causing swallowing or aspiration. In the process of using pusher, fingers should be used to protect soft tissue,

and the fulcrum should be stable to prevent oral mucosa from damaging.

4. A case of early loss of the first deciduous molar, for teeth with tighter interdental space, especially during the eruption of the first permanent molar, the band ring to the second deciduous molar is not easy to be positioned in the case. The dividing ring can be used to separate the teeth, and then the band ring can be tried again after 3 or 5 days.
5. When making a loop, it should be noted that the width of the loop should be enough to allow the eruption of permanent teeth, and should not be an obstacle to prevent the eruption of permanent teeth; loop should be kept at a distance of 0.5 mm from the tissue surface, to avoid the formation of ulcers by compressing the tissue surface.
6. Notify periodic review every 6 months.

Process assessment for students' practice

The instructor will grade the students' practice according to:

- Proper fitting of band rings;
- Careful protection for the tissue surface;
- Proper trimming and polishing for the band;
- Neat final adhesion and proper occlusion.

References

[1] Simon T, Nwabueze I, Oueis H, et al. Space maintenance in the primary and mixed dentitions [J]. Journal of the Michigan Dental Association, 2012, 94 (1): 38-40.

[2] Cernei ER, Maxim DC, Zetu IN. The influence of premature loss of temporary upper molars on permanent molars [J]. Rev Med Chir Soc Med Nat Iasi, 2015, 119 (1): 236-242.

[3] Soxman JA. Handbook of clinical techniques in pediatric dentistry [M]. Shenyang: Liaoning Science and Technology Press, 2017.

CHAPTER 9

APPLIANCES FOR CORRECTION ANTERIOR CROSSBITE IN THE PRIMARY DENTITION

Introduction

Upper removable appliances (URAs) can effectively help to push teeth labially for correcting the anterior crossbites. Anterior crossbites occur when the mandible displaces forward on closure. It seems that URAs can push single or blocks of teeth to be "over the bite". Compared with fixed appliances, such kind of appliance boosts the advantage of incorporating the posterior bite blocks for opening the bite as well as removing all obstacles to the movement of the lower teeth. The spring design changes based on the type of teeth to be moved, a tooth in buccal segment or an incisor. Z-spring is designed for canines and incisors and T-spring for molars and premolars, considering its best fitness to palatal surfaces. Expansion screws can serve for moving blocks of teeth, and a re-curved spring or "double Z-spring" can serve for moving teeth with the same movement direction.

Under the condition that the anterior crossbite can be affected by the mandible's anterior displacement on closure, the elimination of crossbite will lead to the increase in overjet. It is necessary to warn patient together with their parents about such possibility.

Sometimes a displacement on closure can be hard or impossible to detect, considering patients' habit of avoiding premature occlusal contact. The wear of incisor edge shows the possibility of a displacement. However, if there is any doubt, it is the best to assume that no displacement occurs on closure.

Classification

Use of Z-springs

- **Indications**

It is required to push single tooth labially for correcting the anterior crossbite in patients with mandible anterior displacement on closure and/or gingival recession exists on the labial side of the lower tooth that is involved in such crossbite.

Such kind of gingival recession acts as a common result of the anterior crossbite. On that account, it is necessary to assume that a mandibular displacement occurs when a young patient present gingival recession, except as otherwise noted.

- **Contraindications**

There is no displacement of the mandible.

There is minimal or no overbite at the start of treatment.

The teeth to be moved labially are already proclined.

Figure 9 – 1 shows appliance with Z-springs.

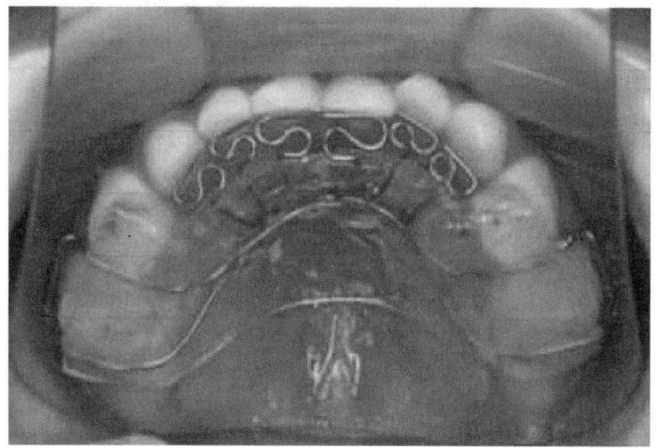

Figure 9 – 1 Appliance with Z-springs.

Use of an expansion screw to move a block of teeth labially

- **Indications**

Correcting anterior crossbite will involve three-to-four incisor teeth.

Rationale: Under such situation, it is necessary to carefully assess teeth prior to treatment because Class Ⅲ skeletal discrepancy may exist potentially. URA can be applied to treatment only in following cases:

- A mandible presents an anterior displacement from edge to edge incisor.
- The overbite is enough for ensuring that the correction is stable.
- The upper incision is not proclined or the lower incisor is not retroclined, both of them demonstrate the dental compensation for an obviously potential skeletal discrepancy.

- **Contraindications**

There is no displacement of the mandible.

There is minimal or no overbite at the start of treatment.

The teeth to be moved labially are already proclined.

The teeth to be moved require labial movement but in different directions. A screw appliance will move the block of teeth in one direction only, which may not be appropriate.

Figure 9 – 2 shows appliance with expansion screws.

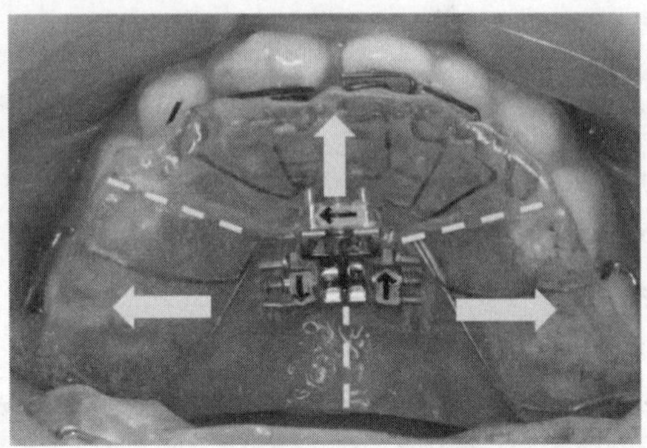

Figure 9 – 2 Appliance with expansion screws.

The objective of lab practice

1. To know Indications and contraindications of the URAs.
2. To know design features of a URA to correct an anterior crossbite of the upper incisor teeth.

Materials and instruments

Figure 9 – 3 demonstrates some of the materials and instruments for making the URA.

1. Stainless steel wire 0.7 mm.
2. Young loop bending plier.
3. Prong plier.
4. Adams plier.
5. Wire cutter.
6. Marking pencil.
7. Polymer or powder resin.
8. Denture base polymer liquid.

Components description

- **retentive components**

In general, retentive components are wire clasps, and the most common components are Adams's clasps (also called "universal" clasps as they are applied to posterior teeth or anterior teeth) and Southend clasps (applied to one or two adjacent anterior teeth). The Adams clasps is composed of arrow heads, bridges and retentive parts. Sometimes retentive components can be C-clasps or other types of labial bow, with the latter widely used to retain appliances thus also called retainers. There are also other types but they are not often used.

- **acrylic baseplate**

Acrylic baseplate will not be modified under passive appliance, while it may include a bite plane or posterior capping under active appliances.

- **active components**

Active component refers to wire springs in most cases, screws in special cases and labial bow in rare cases, but it is suggested to dismiss bows specific to active tooth movement under most circumstance considering the limited indication. When using URA to tip teeth, it is required to apply light forces (25 – 50 g, 50 g maximum) per spring.

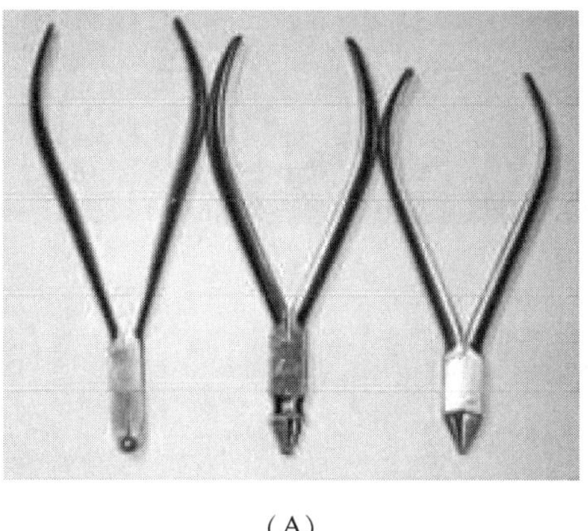

(A)

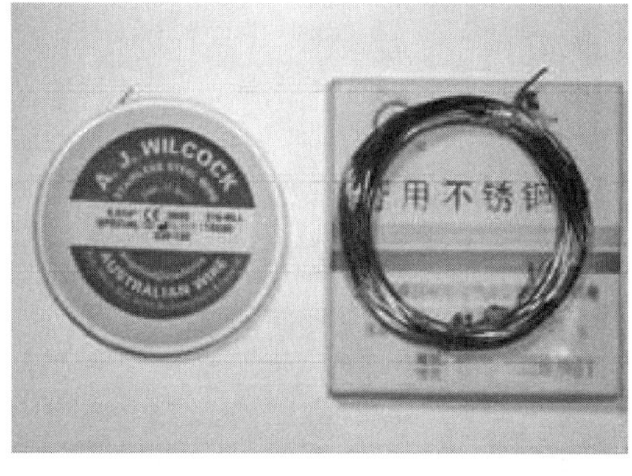

(B)

Figure 9 – 3 Materials and instruments.

Practice steps

- **Adams's clasps on 55, 65, 16, 26**

The Adams's clasp should be made of 0.7 mm hard stainless steel wire for all teeth except canines or which 0.6 mm is preferred.

- Fabricated with 0.7 mm wire engaging the mesio-buccal and disto-buccal undercuts of the posterior teeth.
- Usually placed on first molars.
- Does not tend to separate the teeth when it is clasping.
- The mesial and distal undercuts of the molar are marked on the cast. The distance between

these two marks would form the length of the bridge of the Adams.

- 0.7 mm hard round stainless steel wire is used. A 90° bend is made (Figure 9 - 4).

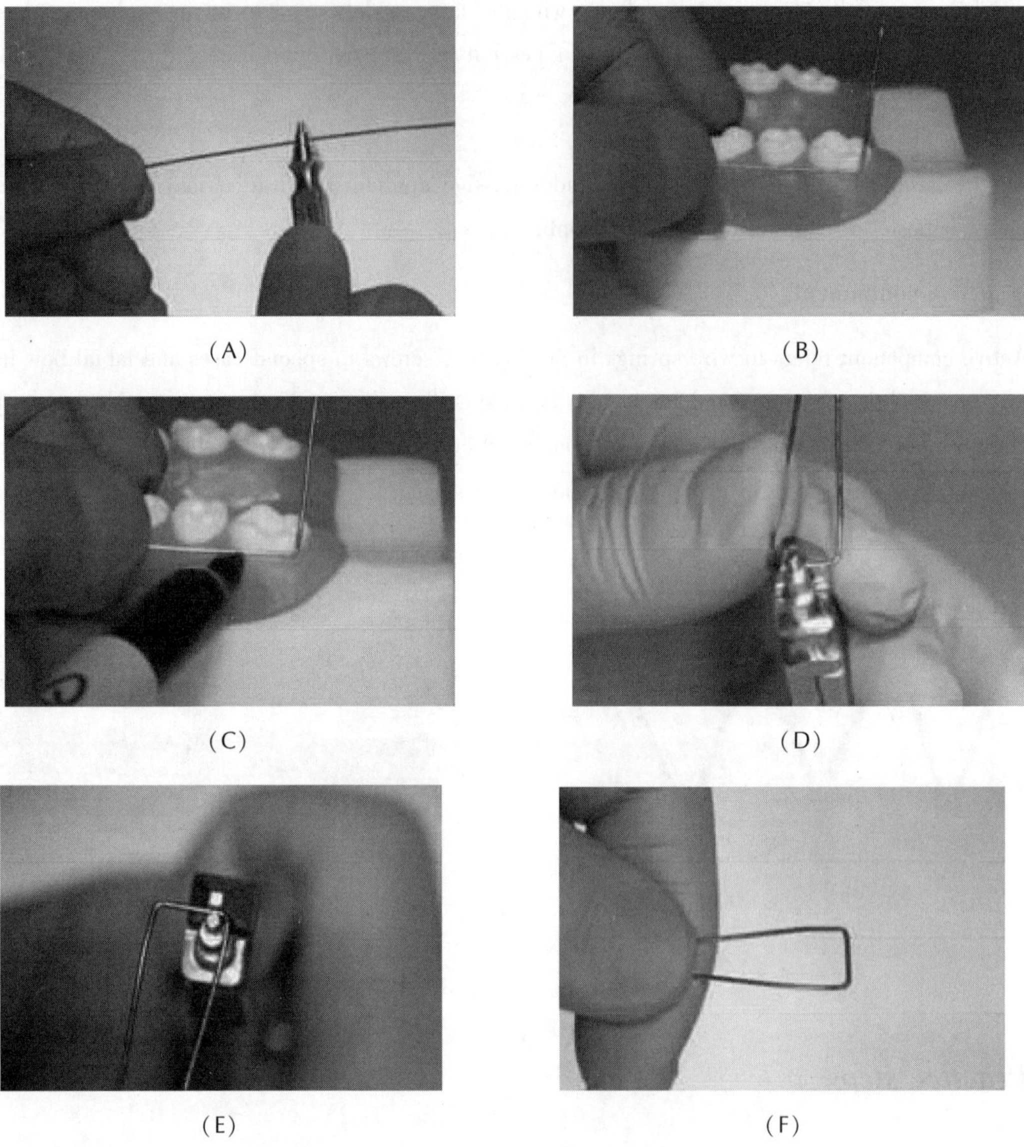

Figure 9 - 4 Adams's clasps (Part 1).

- The formation of the arrowhead. The wire is first bent at right angles.
- The clasp is tilted downwards against the pliers and the arrowhead formed by bending outside the tip of the beak.
- The second arrowhead is formed in the same way. The arrowheads are aligned to follow the contours of the gum.
- The arrowheads are squeezed slightly to make the correct width.
- The clasp is tried on the tooth.

· The arrowhead is grasped from inside the clasp and the tag bent up at 90°.
· The tag is then bent outwards and a further 45° over but not around the tip of the beaks (Figure 9 −5, Figure 9 −6).
· The clasp is tried on the tooth.
· The tag is completed. The second tag is completed in the same way (Figure 9 −7).

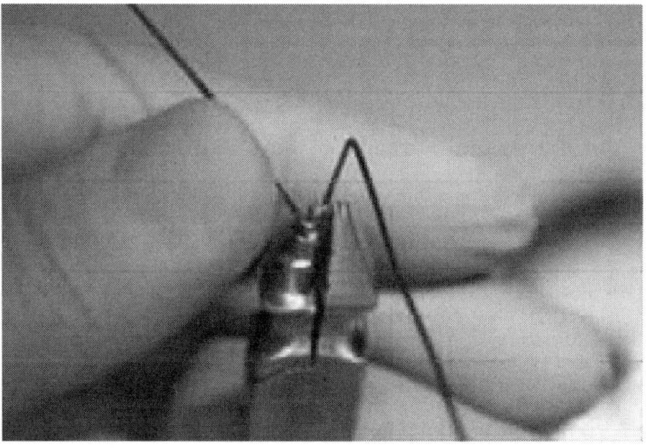

Figure 9 −5 Adams's clasps (Part 2).

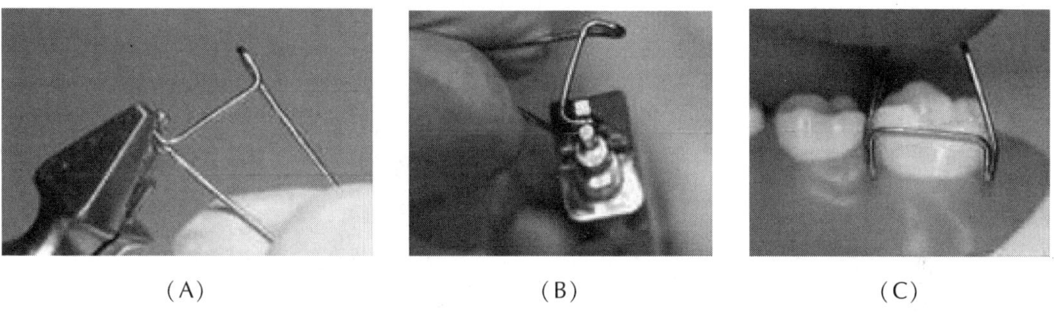

(A) (B) (C)

Figure 9 −6 Adams's clasps (Part 3).

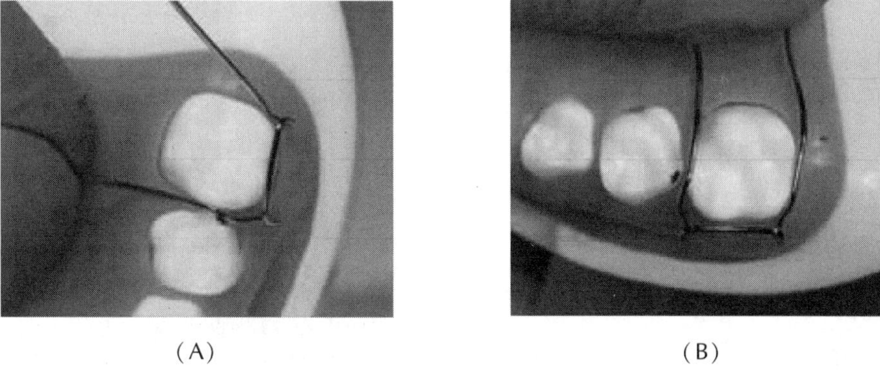

(A) (B)

Figure 9 −7 Adams clasps (Part 4).

- **Acrylic base (optional practice)**

· The model is prepared by removing bubbles in palatal gingival area. After sharpening all margins and making space for the arrow clasps, paint the model with a separating medium.

- This method is called increment method or drop and powder method.
- All wire parts are added to cast.
- Now add the polymer or powder resin in increments to palatal surface of cast and then monomer, start spreading it slowly. A thickness of 2 mm is acquired.

- **Z-springs**

It has two helices and resembles the shape of "Z."

- Adapt 0.5 mm wire on the palatal surfaces of the teeth to be proclined and place a helix at one of its ends.
- Adapt the wire parallel to the active arm and place another helix at the far end of first helix within the limit of the tooth.
- Form the second helix adapt the wire parallel to the active arm.
- Use Young loop bending plier close the Z-springs up or down.
- At mid-point place a right-angled bend and then place a vertical bend towards the palatal side so that spring is positioned perpendicular to the cingulum.
- Adapt continuously to form a retentive tag (Figure 9 - 8).

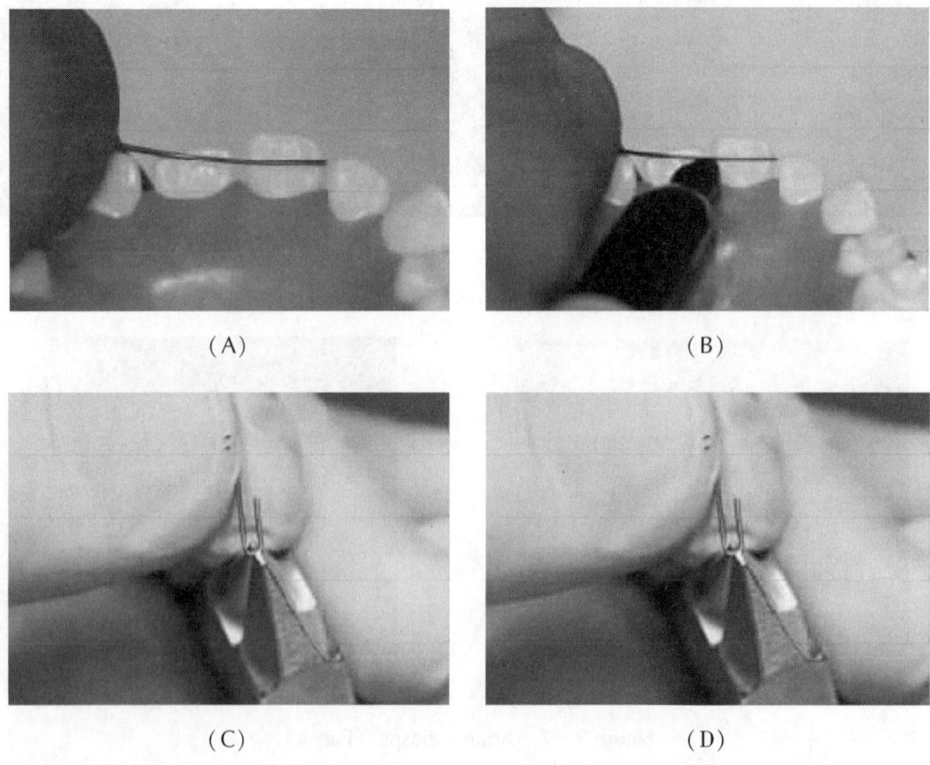

(A) (B)

(C) (D)

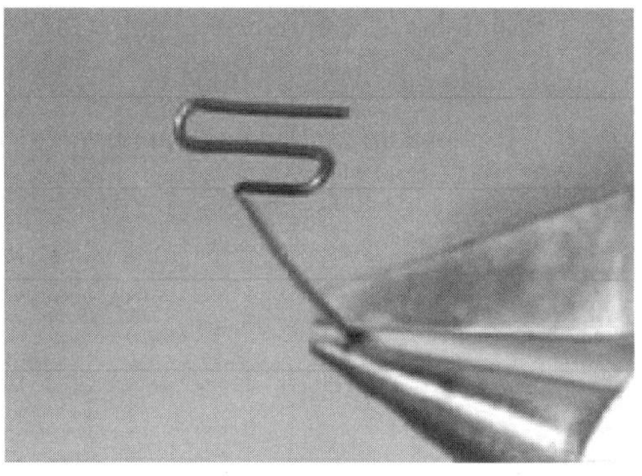

(E)

Figure 9 –8 Z-spring.

Process assessment for students' practice

- **Adams's clasps**

· The fly-over should be as close to the contact points of the teeth as possible as they cross from the palatal acrylic to the buccal aspect of the teeth.

· The bridge should lie approximately two-thirds of the distance from the gingival margin to the cusp tips, and there should be a gap of no more than 1.5 mm between the bridge and the buccal surface of the tooth.

· The arrowheads should be positioned in the undercuts just above the gingival margins on the mesio-buccal and disto-buccal aspects of the crown.

- **Z-springs**

It's important that the free arm of the Z-springs lies parallel to the palatal surface of the tooth to ensure even contact and, hence, even force distribution on the tooth. Point contact on the palatal surface will induce rotational movements.

- **Acrylic base**

· The baseplate should be checked for closeness of fit with the palate.

· The baseplate should also be checked to ensure that no acrylic will prevent the planned movement of teeth.

References

[1] Luther F. Orthodontic retainers and removable appliances [M]. Oxford: Wiley-Blackwell, 2013.

[2] Veis RB, Christian JC. Principles of appliance therapy for adults and children [M]. Charsworth, CA: Appliance Therapy Group, 2004.

[3] Graber TM, Neumann B. Removable orthodontic appliances [M]. Philadelphia: W. B. Saunders Co., 1984.

CHAPTER 10

MANUFACTURE OF MAXILLARY SPACE-REGAINING APPLIANCE

Introduction of maxillary expansion and Coffin Spring Maxillary expander

Expansion have been used to correct maxillary transverse deficiency for more than a century. The main objective of maxillary expansion is correcting transverse discrepancy between maxillary and mandibular arch, especially for crossbite in posterior teeth. There are three modalities for maxillary expansion today: rapid maxillary expansion (RME), slow maxillary expansion (SME), and surgically assisted maxillary expansion.

RME

The aim of RME is to open the maxillary suture with heavy force and minimize the tipping movement of posterior teeth. The RME appliance consists of banded and bonded appliances. The banded appliances are welded to the bands on maxillary first molars and first premolars. The bonded appliances are constructed with an acrylic cap which is bonded directly to the maxillary teeth.

SME

SME produce less force on the maxillary bone and teeth. It has been found to have greater post-expansion stability after an adequate retention time. There are several appliances for SME: Coffin spring, Magnets, W-arch, Quahelix and so on.

Surgically assisted maxillary expansion

Surgically assisted maxillary expansion is suitable for the skeletally mature patients, who need the correction of maxillary transverse deficiency. There are two techniques available: surgically assisted rapid palatal expansion and segmental maxillary surgery.

There are so many appliances for maxillary expansion. Neither RME nor surgically assisted maxillary expansion is suitable for practice in laboratory. Coffin spring appliances was described by Walter H. Coffin in 1881. It is an effective appliance for slow maxillary expansion. In this chapter, the manufacture procedure of Coffin spring appliances will be introduced.

The objective of lab practice

1. To master how to make a Coffin spring.
2. To master how to make Adams's clasps.
3. To be familiar with the construction of baseplates with self-curing acrylic resins.
4. To know the procedure of trimming and polishing removable appliance.

Materials and instruments

1. 1.0 mm stainless steel wire [Figure 10 - 1 (A)].
2. 0.7 mm stainless steel wire [Figure 10 - 1 (A)].
3. Self-curing acrylic powder and liquid [Figure 10 - 1 (B)].
4. Young loop forming pliers [Figure 10 - 1 (C)].

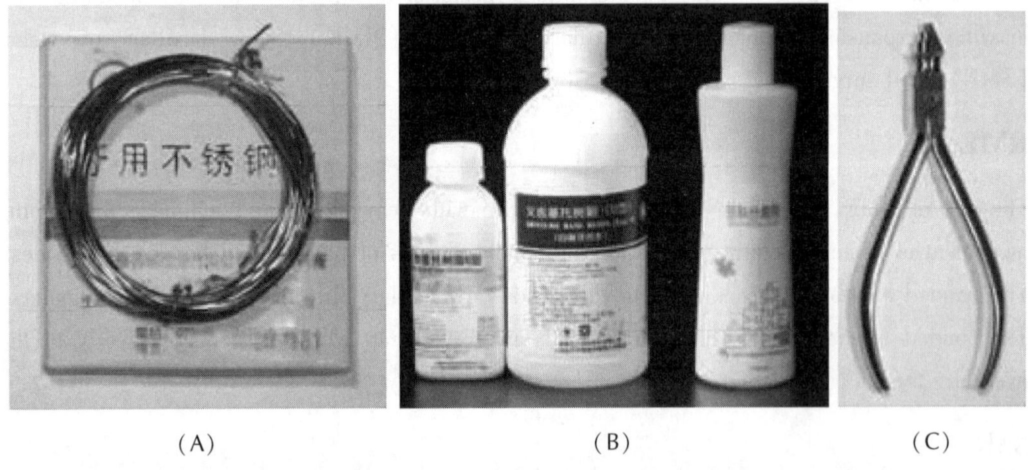

(A) (B) (C)

Figure 10 - 1 Materials and instruments.

Practice steps

1. The model should be inspected and trimmed to allow the Adams's clasps to engage the undercuts.
2. The wire for Coffin spring is 1.0 mm thick stainless steel round wire. A diamond-shape or a generous loop is formed in the center with pliers, it stands 1.0 mm away from the palatal roof (Figure 10 - 2).

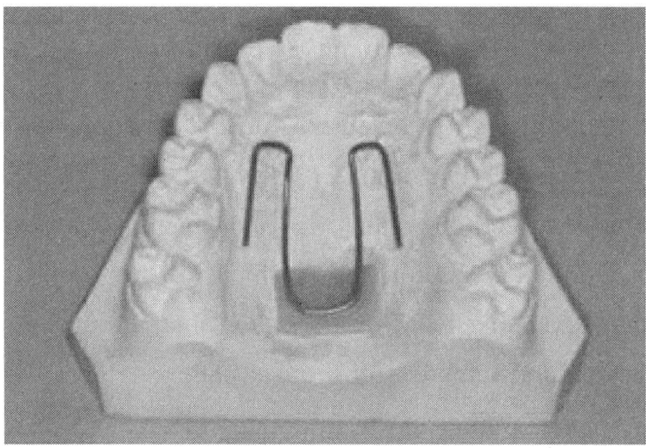

Figure 10 -2　Coffin spring.

3. Adams's clasps are most constructed with 0.7mm hard stainless steel round wire. The construction steps include:

- Define the bridge of the clasp by bending the wire to a little beyond a right angle at each end [Figure 10 -3 (A)].

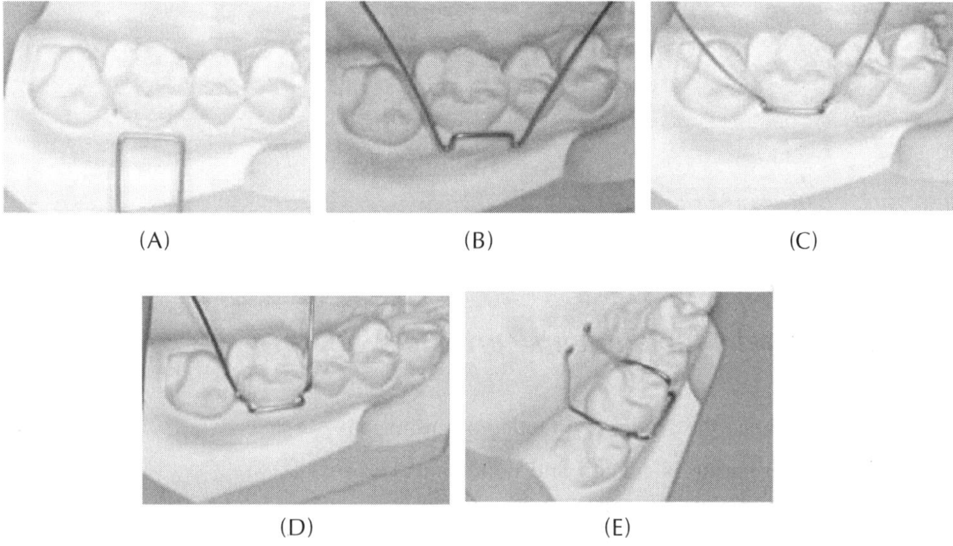

(A)　(B)　(C)　(D)　(E)

Figure 10 -3　Adams's clasps.

- The ends of the wire are bent up to form the arrowheads. The bends is best made over the tips of plier to make sure a sufficiently narrow head [Figure 10 -3 (B)].
- Bend the arrowheads to an angle of around 45° to the bridge to permit the arrowheads sit correctly against the tooth [Figure 10 -3 (C)].
- The arrowheads sit at about 45° to the long axis of the tooth and the outer arm of the arrowhead should be bent through around 90° so that the free end will rest across the embrasure when the clasp is correctly positioned [Figure 10 -3 (D)].
- Finish off the tags. Each tag should be not traumatized by the opposing teeth. [Figure 10 -

3 (E)].

- Bend four Adams's clasps on the first premolars and first molars.

4. Both heat-curing and self-curing acrylic resins can be used for construction of baseplates. Here takes the self-curing acrylic resin for example. First the clasps and springs are positioned correctly on the teeth by pink wax and coated with a film of the appropriate separating material. The parts of Coffin spring which will not be bound up in the baseplate are covered with pink wax. Mixed the resin powder and liquid then apply the resin to the model. Modify the shape and thickness of the baseplate.
5. Trim and polish the appliance after the resin cured (Figure 10 -4).

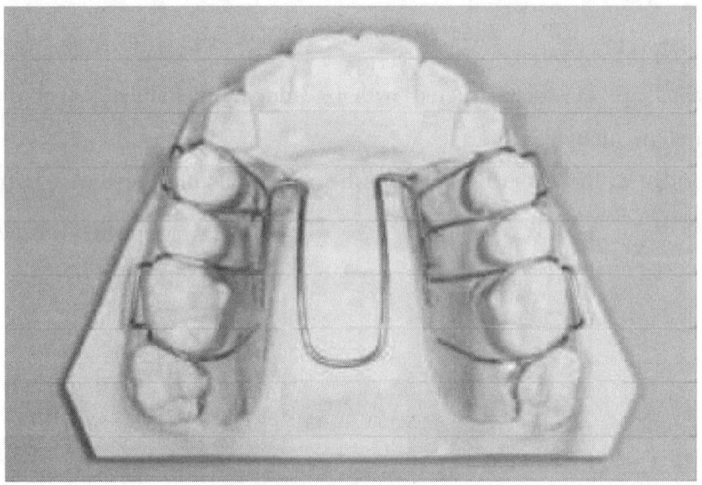

Figure 10 -4 Coffin Spring appliance.

Process assessment for students' practice

The instructor will grades the students' practice according to:

1. The bent of Coffin spring is smooth and no obvious crease.
2. Proper bent of Adams' clasps and no traumatization to the opposing teeth.
3. The proper shape and polishing of baseplate and surface.

References

[1] Proffit WR, Fields HW, Larson BE, et al. Contemporary orthodontics [M], 6th ed. Amesterdam: Elsevier, 2013.

[2] Philipandams C. The Design, Construction & use of removable orthodontic appliances [M]. 5th ed. Bristol: John Wright & Sons, 1984.

CHAPTER 11

OROFACIAL MUSCLE TRAINING FOR ORAL HABITS

Background of the orofacial muscle training

Equilibrium Considerations in occlusion

The dentition is in an equilibrium status which is the basic theory for orofacial muscle training. The teeth are subjected to various forces such as lip, tongue, masticatory muscles, swallowing and speaking efforts, but do not move under usual circumstances. When orthodontic movement happens, the teeth and PDL needs light force of long duration (6 hours or so per day). It means if the balance between long-duration pressure from the tongue versus lip or cheek pressure changes, the tooth movement will happen.

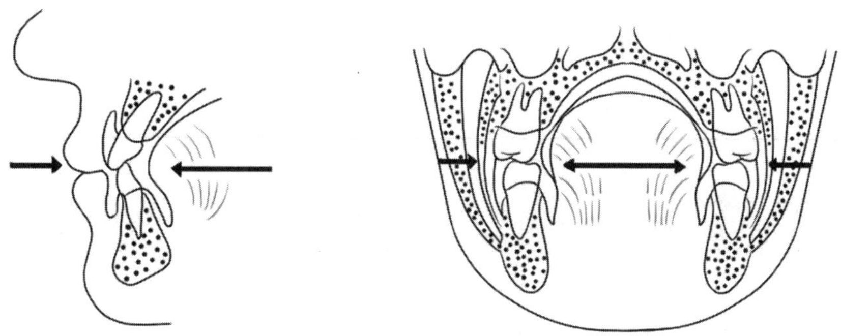

Figure 11 −1 Equilibrium theory.

The influence of deleterious oral habits on occlusion

Previous researches (Brandhorst, 1932) showed 25% of the etiologies which cause malocclusion, are deleterious oral habits. Also researches in Japan showed 40% malocclusions in primary dentition are related to deleterious oral habits. If the oral habits are intercepted before 2. 5 − 3 years by teaching method, most of the malocclusions can be self-correcting. However, if the deleterious oral habits persist beyond the time that the permanent teeth begin to erupt, malocclusion will occur.

- **Digital sucking**

Digital sucking will cause deep overjet or open bite. When a child places a thumb in the mouth, the thumb will press lingually against the lower incisor and labially against the upper incisors. Meanwhile, the cheek pressure increases when sucking and low positioned tongue decreases the pressure against upper posterior teeth, along causes a narrow upper arch. Sometimes, children suck index finger or middle finger, the malocclusion will change to crossbite, labially positioned lower incisors or partial open bite as the finger positioned angle changes. Intermittent sucking may not displace the incisor, but those who suck thumb or finger over 6 hours a day, particularly sucking while sleeping, can cause a significant malocclusion.

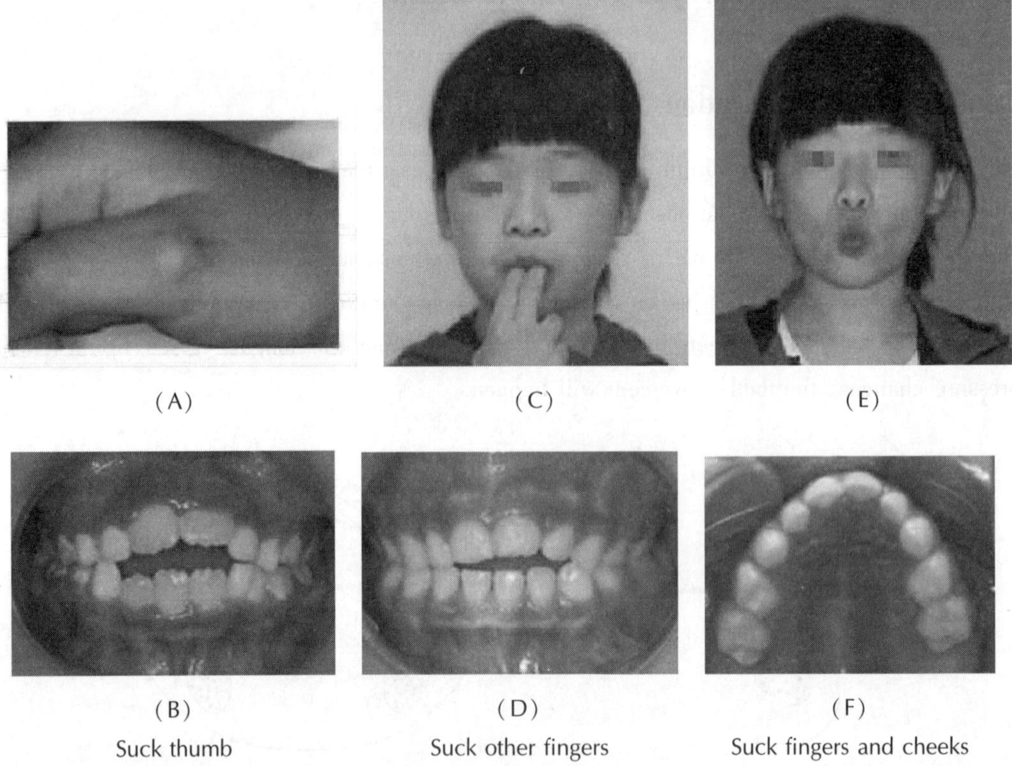

Figure 11 −2　Digital sucking habit.

(A) and (B): Thumb sucking will cause spindle shaped open bite of the anterior teeth or deep overjet, sometimes callus can be found on the thumb. (C) and (D): Sucking index finger or middle finger may cause partial open bite or crossbite of the anterior teeth. (E) and (F): Sucking cheeks will cause narrow upper arch, and may resulted in posterior teeth crossbite.

Digital sucking is also associated with open bite especially evolved in normal eruption of incisors and excessive eruption of posterior teeth. When a thumb or a finger is placed between the teeth, the incisors eruption is directly impeded. The separation of the jaws causes more eruption of the posterior teeth at the same time, thus develop an anterior open bite (Figure 11 -2).

- **Lip biting habit**

How lip biting habit influence the occlusion differs from biting upper lip or biting lower lip. Biting habit changes the pressure of the lip on the teeth, and causes overjet or crossbite. When biting lower lip, the pressure of the lower lip against lower incisors increases, while upper incisors receive more labial pressure from displaced lower lip at the same time, flared upper incisors and lingually inclined lower incisor would be the result. The pressure on the jaw also keep the mandible on a recession position, further aggravate the Class Ⅱ malocclusion. On the contrary, biting upper lip can cause crossbite and Class Ⅲ malocclusion (Figure 11 -3).

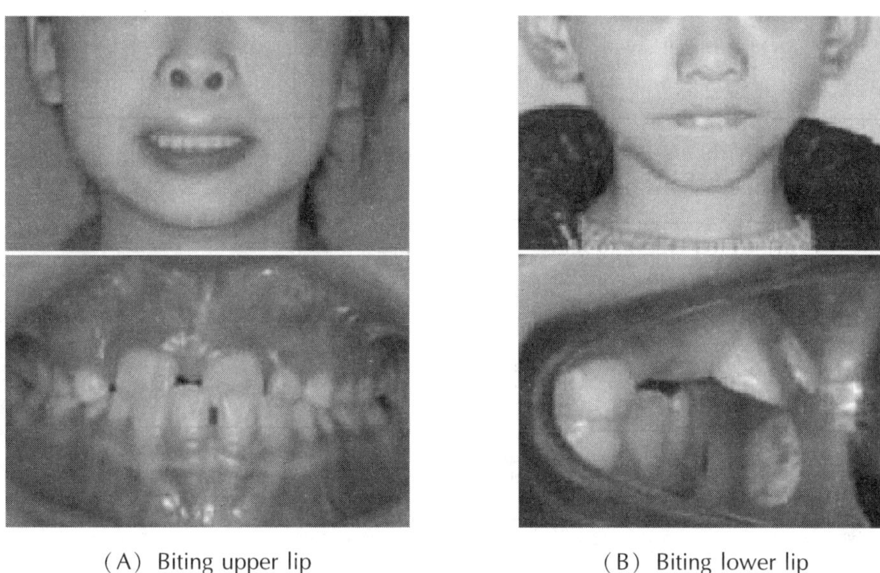

(A) Biting upper lip (B) Biting lower lip

Figure 11 -3 Results of biting upper lip (A) and biting lower lip (B).

- **Tongue thrust swallow**

A tongue thrust swallow is more likely to be the result of displaced incisors and as a physiologic adaption, not the cause. It is neither necessary nor desirable to try to teach the patient to swallow differently before beginning orthodontic treatment. However, tongue tip protrusion during swallowing is sometimes associated with a forward tongue posture. If a patient has a forward resting posture of the tongue, the duration of the light pressure between the anterior tooth could affect tooth position, vertically or horizontally, and will aggravate existed open bite. Protrusion of the incisors, anterior open bite, molar occlusal increase and lower facial height increase are related malocclusions that may caused by tongue thrust swallow pattern (Figure 11 - 4 and Figure 11 -5).

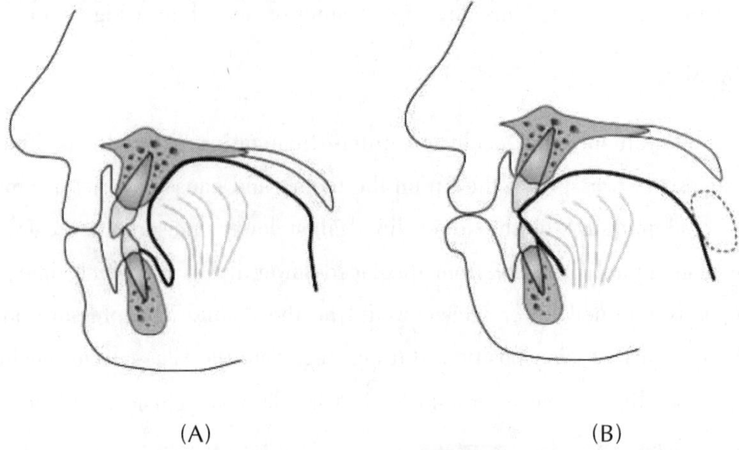

(A) (B)

Figure 11 －4 (A): Normal swallowing: The masticatory muscles play a role in making the upper and lower teeth tightly bite, and maintain this state during the whole swallowing process. Then lips relax, the tongue tip places against the palatal roof behind the upper incisors, and the posterior teeth brought into occlusion during swallowing. (b): Abnormal swallowing: The tongue often moves forward, positioned between the upper and lower incisors, forming a tongue swallowing. The tip of the tongue is between the anterior teeth, or against the lower incisor when swallowing.

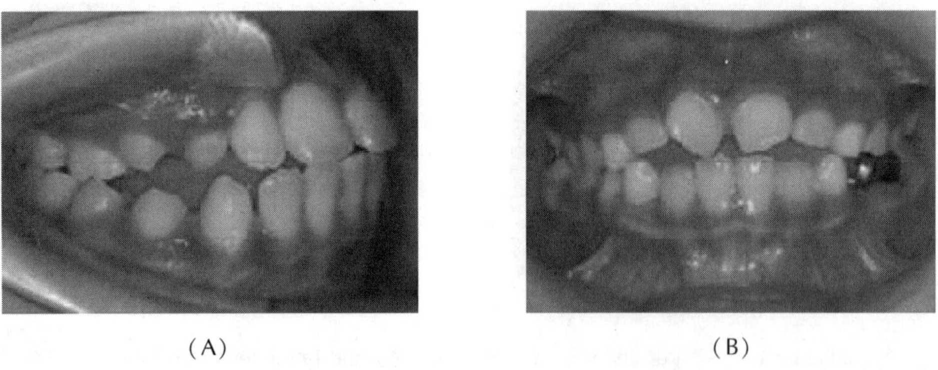

(A) (B)

Figure 11 －5 Protrusion of the incisors (A) or anterior open bite (B) may be caused by tongue thrust habits.

• Mouth breathing/Respiratory pattern

Mouth breathing is associated with malocclusions characterized by deep overjet, a narrow upper dental arch, mandibular retrusion and vertical increase of the facial height as it in turn alters the equilibrium of pressures on the jaws, teeth arch, cheek and tongue. Three effects on growth would be expected when mouth breathing:

- anterior face height would increase, and posterior teeth would super-erupt.
- unless there was unusual vertical growth of the ramus, the mandible would rotate down and back, opening the bite anteriorly and increasing overjet.
- increased pressure from the stretched cheeks might cause a narrower maxillary dental arch.

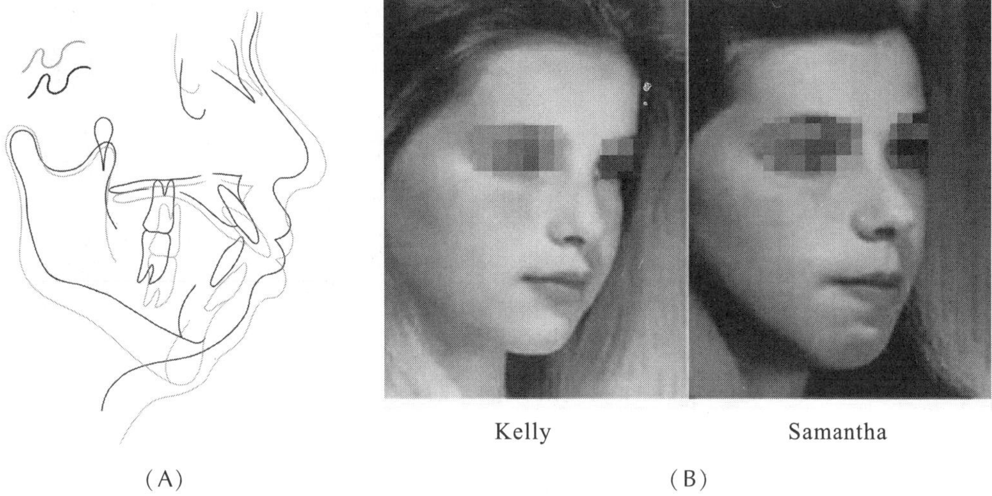

(A) (B)

Figure 11 -6 (A): Cephalometric superimposition showing the effect of mouth. breathing From age 12 (black) to 16 (grey), we can find that the mandible obviously rotated downward and backward during growth (Redraw from McNamara JA. Angle Orthod. 1981 (51): 269 -300). (B) Different twins profile after adenoidectomy with nose breathing (Kelly) and with mouth breathing (Samantha). (McKeown P, Mew J. Cranio-facial changes and mouth breathing [J]. Irish Dental J, 2011, 57 (3): 12 -18, 17).

The objective of lab practice

1. To master checkup of the deleterious oral habits and corresponding muscle training.
2. To be familiar with the appliances that will be used in the treatment.

Materials and instruments

1. Tissue paper [Figure 11 -7 (A)].
2. Buttons over 30 mm diameter and cotton thread [Figure 11 -7 (B)].
3. Hardboard or plastic board [Figure 11 -7 (C)].
4. Chewing gum [Figure 11 -7 (D)].

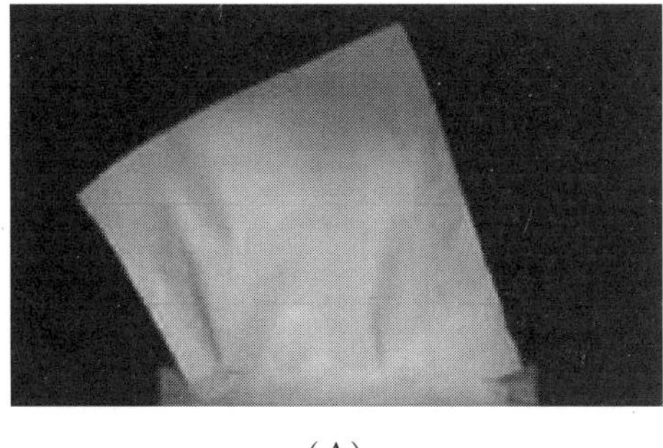

(A)

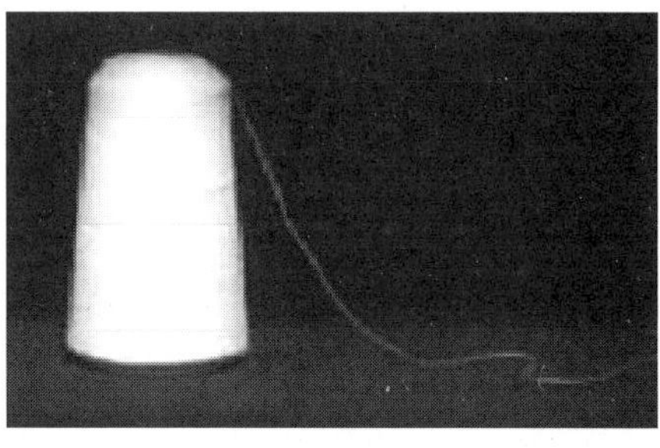

(B)

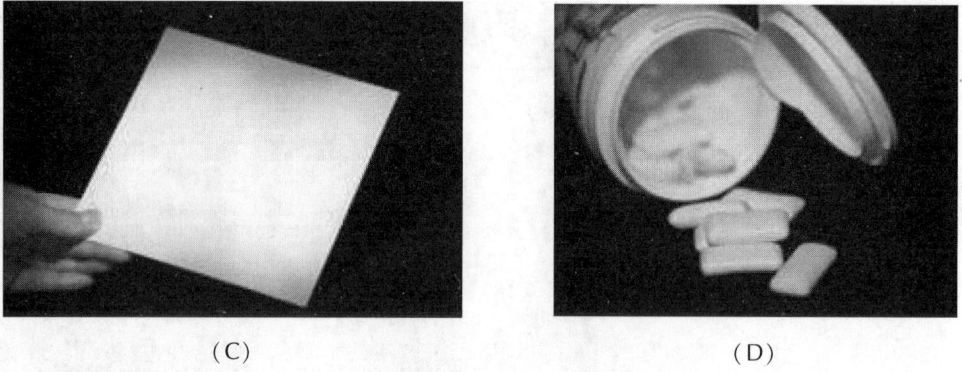

(C) (D)

Figure 11 –7 Materials and instruments.

Practice steps

1. Group practice: follow the teacher's instruction and be familiar with each orofacial muscle training.
2. Performing part: each group will perform a kind of deleterious oral habits, other groups will play the "doctor" to checkup and direct the "patients" to do orofacial muscle training.

Clinic checkup of deleterious oral habits

Before clinic checkup, one should communicate with the parents for enough time, and collect information from the parents such as mouth breathing during sleep or other habits when child feels anxious.

Deleterious oral habits should be observed when a child is familiar with the clinic environment. Indeed, deleterious oral habits usually happen when children are anxious or insecure, but dental checkup will give anxieties to children which may lead children to do some posture or behavior they usually not do, especially some habits like lip biting or digital sucking. Dentists can quietly observe the child when talking with parents, then do oral checkup when child is familiar with the dental chair, dentists and clinic environment. Severe digital sucking can cause callus on the thumb. Mouth breathing can be easily observed when a child has nasal obstruction, but sometimes the child can close the lip consciously and conceal the diagnosis. A hydroncus line on the cheek can be observed when a child has sucking cheek habit (Figure 11 – 8 to Figure 11 – 10).

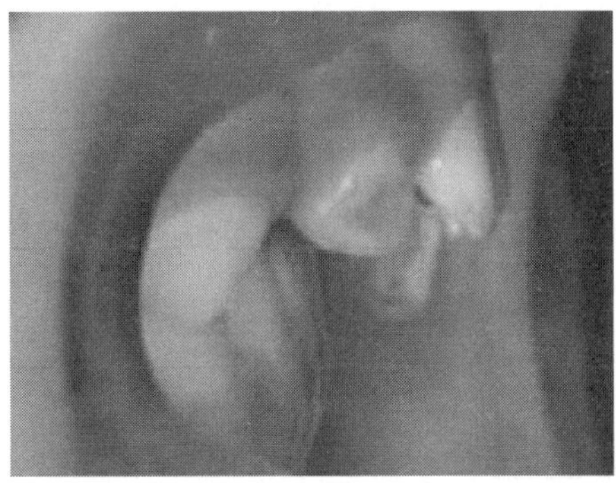
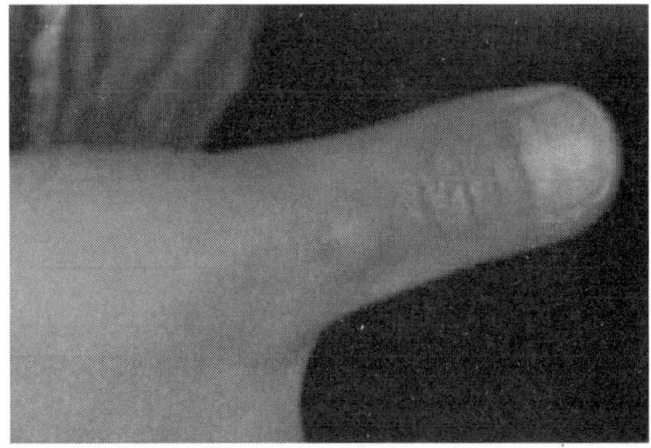

Figure 11 −8 Deep overjet and callus caused by digital sucking.

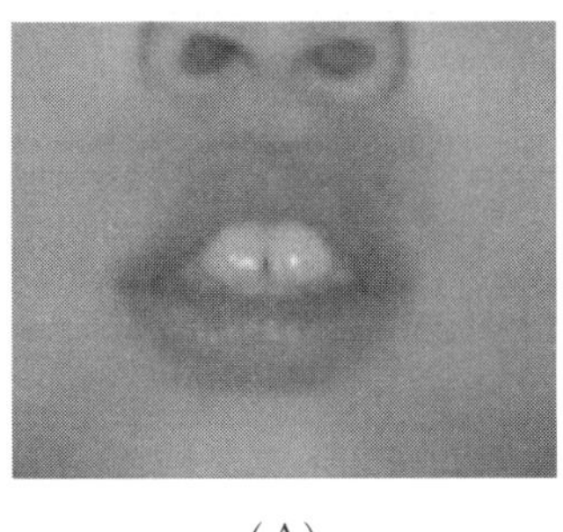
(A)

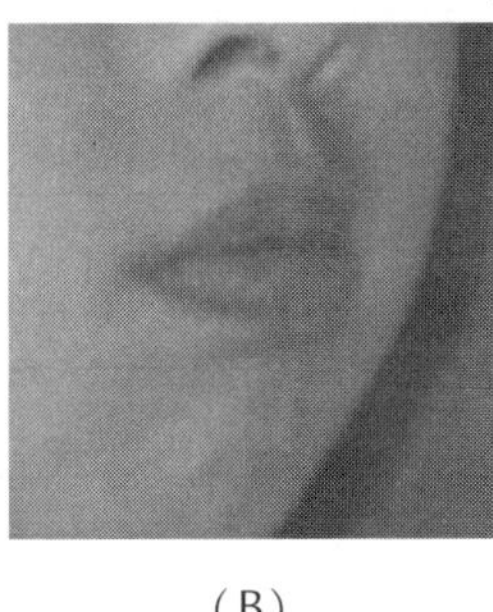
(B)

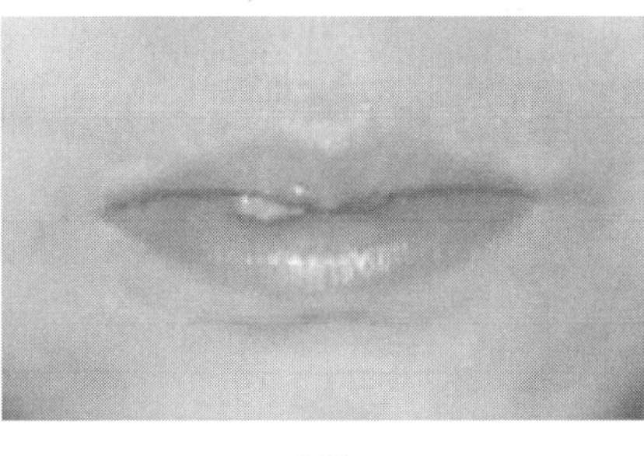
(C)

Figure 11 − 9 (A) and (B) A child with mouth breathing, and can only close the lip by constriction of the Orbicularis oris muscle, (C) A child can close the lip consciously.

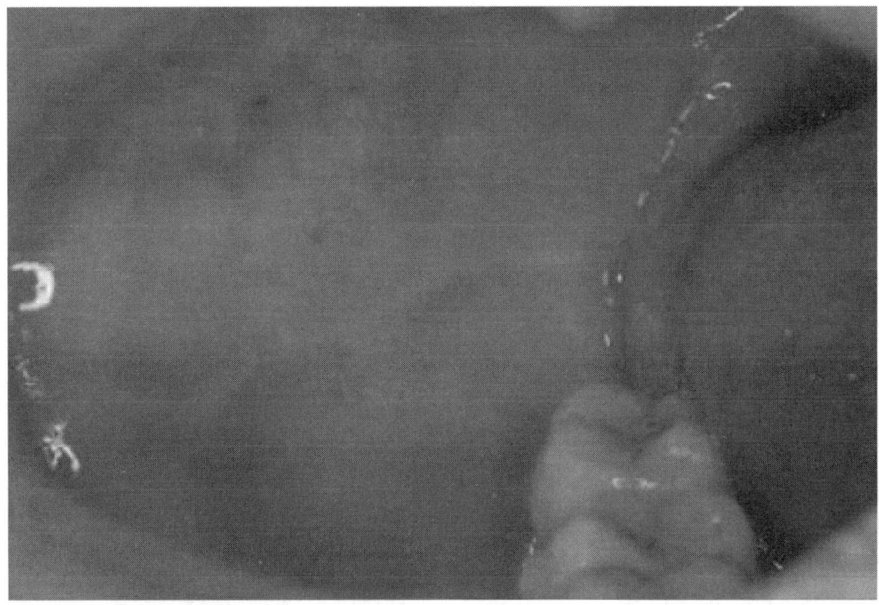

Figure 11 −10 A hydroncus line on the cheek when sucking cheeks.

Interceptive of the deleterious oral habits

Teaching by the parents and dentist is first recommended. The children must be willing to correct the oral habits and have compliance to wear the appliances or do myofunction treatment, otherwise the interceptive treatment is useless. The following Table 11 - 1 lists possible appliances for each deleterious oral habits, please note these appliances should be used when treating malocclusion and some appliances can be used together.

Table 11 - 1 Possible appliances for each deleterious oral habits.

Digital sucking	Lip bar, Vestibular shield, Tongue thorn
Lip biting	Vestibular shield, Frankel, lip bumper, functional appliances
Tongue thrust	Tongue thorn, Frankel Ⅳ with tongue thorn, maxillary expansion with tongue thorn
Mouth breathing	Nasal obstruction problem should be referred to an otolaryngologist. Malocclusion caused by mouth breathing should be treated according to the specific clinic appearance, usually functional appliances, maxillary expansion appliances can be used

Orofacial muscle training

One should be noted, there is no treatment effect to perform myofunction training without correcting malocclusion. Myofunction training is only considered as a preventive method when children have normal occlusion or wearing retainers, or an auxiliary method while treating malocclusion. Myofunction training itself doesn't have any treatment effect on malocclusion.

- **Lip muscle training**

1. Paper-blowing practice (Figure 11 - 11).

Close the upper and lower lips tightly, inhale, and make a plosive sound.

Close the upper and lower lips tightly, and blow quickly to make a "po" sound.

Put a piece of paper in front of you and blow up the paper when you make a "po" sound.

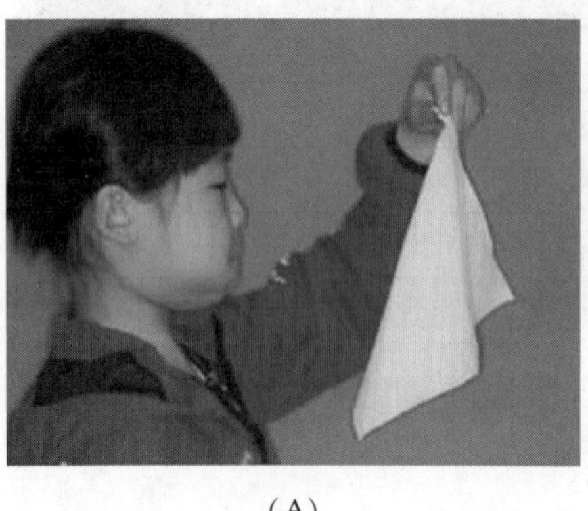

(A)

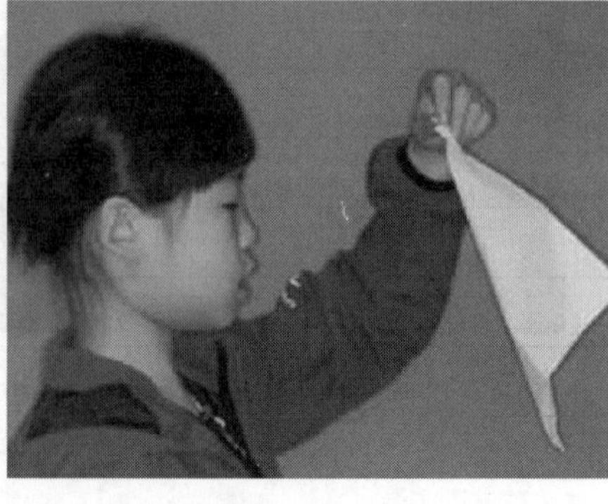

(B)

Figure 11 - 11 Paper-blowing practice.

2. Paper-picking practice (Figure 11 - 12).

Hold a thick paper for more than 15 minutes.

Parents can try to remove the paper while the lips are tightly closed and children try not to let the paper be taken away.

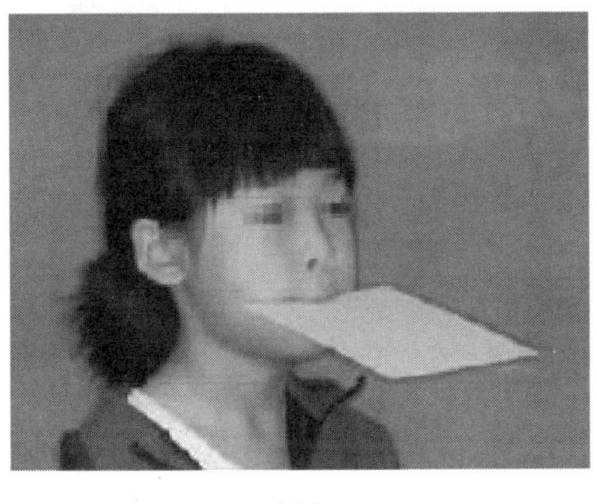

(A)

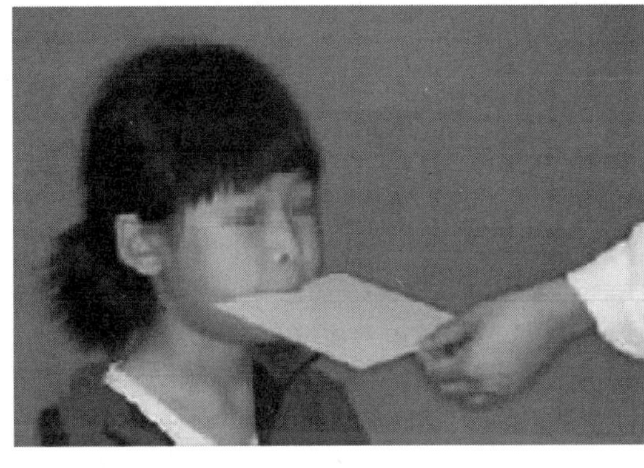

(B)

Figure 11 - 12 Paper-picking practice.

3. Water-holding/Wrapping practice (Figure 11 - 13).

Hold/Wrap a mouthful of water, bow your head, close your lips and slowly let the water flow out.

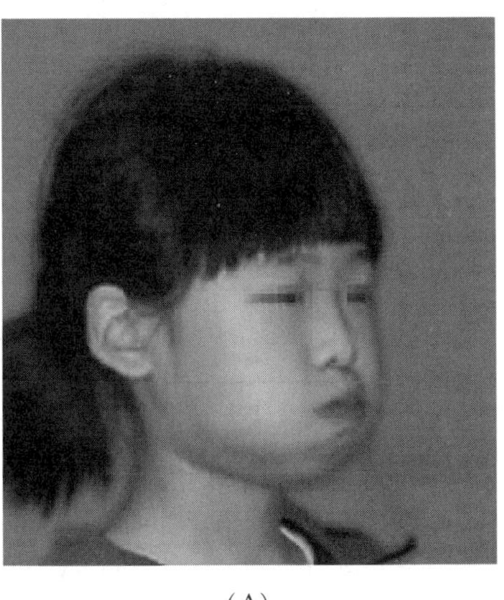

(A)

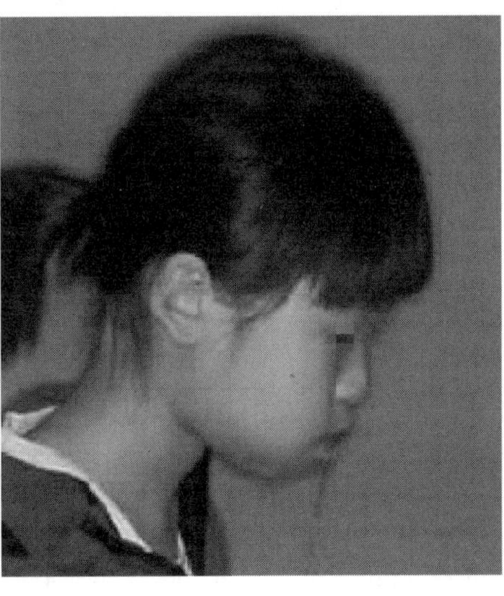

(B)

Figure 11 - 13 Water-holding/wrapping practice.

4. "Eating noodles" practice.

A cotton thread, without teeth, using the lip to simulate eating noodles, "eat" the cotton thread into the mouth.

5. Button practice (Figure 11 - 14).

The button is threaded and placed in the mouth, leaving the thread outside. Pull the thread outward, and the lips wrap the button so that it is not pulled out.

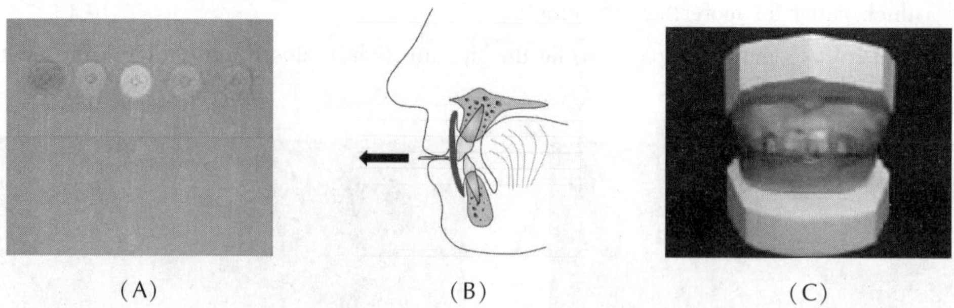

(A) (B) (C)

Figure 11 - 14 Button practice.

- **Tongue muscle training**

1. Tongue-lift and tongue-springing training (Figure 11 - 15).

Step A : If children cannot lift the tongue, we should teach them to find the position of the tip of the tongue when making the "n, t, d" sound firstly.

Step B: When counting "1, 2, 3, 4", the tongue is lifted on the back to hold the hard palate. And then counting "5, 6, 7, 8", make a clicking sound.

Repeat 20 times.

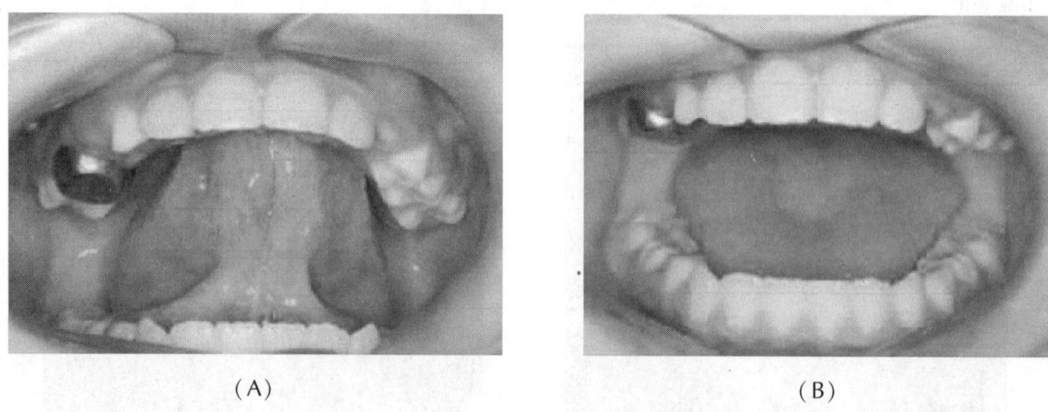

(A) (B)

Figure 11 - 15 Tongue muscle training.

2. Close the upper and lower lips to swallow with the tongue contacting with the palate.

When counting "1, 2, 3, 4", close the upper and lower lips, and the upper and lower teeth gently bite with the tongue contacting with the palate; And then counting "5, 6, 7, 8", swallow saliva.

3. Chewing gum training (Figure 11 - 16).

Step A: Chew the gum into a mass on the tip of the tongue.

Step B: Place the gum on the palate.

Step C: Spread the gum with the tongue to enlarge the area of the gum, swallow and flat the gum at the palate.

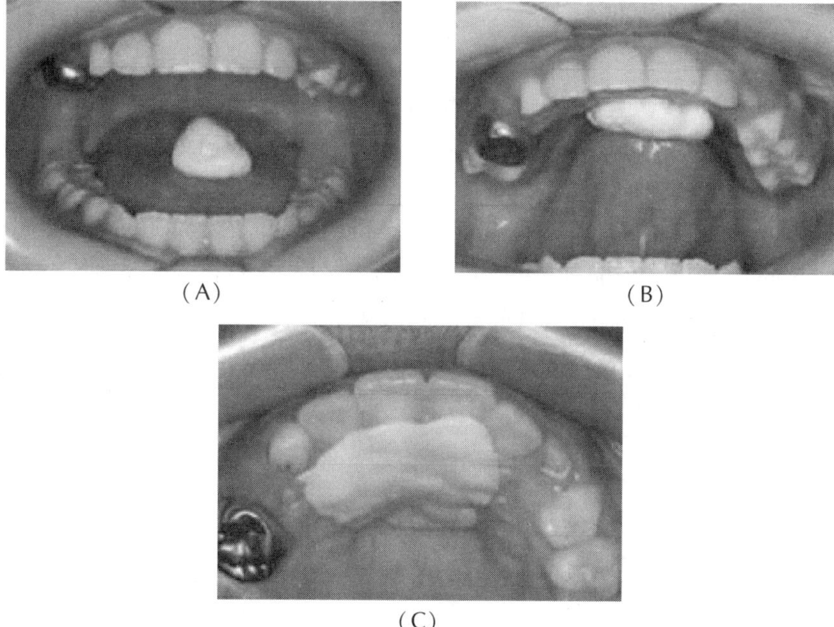

(A) (B) (C)

Figure 11 −16 Chewing gum training.

4. Tongue-rolling training (Figure 11 −17).

Step A: Roll up the tongue, starting from the incisor.

Step B-C: Then roll it back to the junction of soft and hard palate for 5 seconds. 2 rounds per day, 50 times a group.

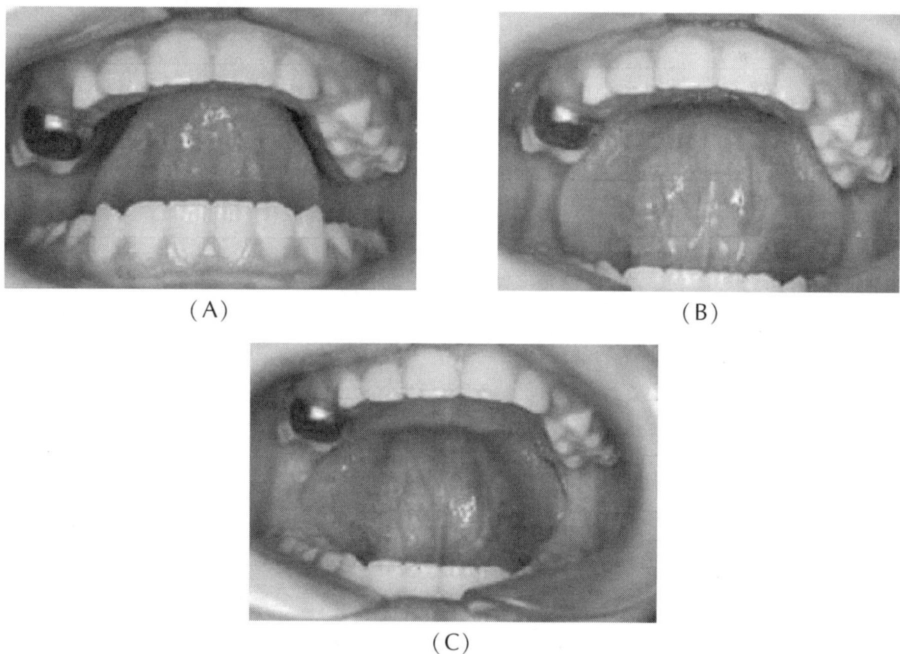

(A) (B) (C)

Figure 11 −17 Tongue-rolling training.

- **Standing Posture training**

Stand against the wall for 5 minutes, with the shoulders naturally drooping, the shoulder blades, the abdominal muscles and the hip muscles tightening (black arrows), and the thigh muscles clamping. Stretch bilateral shoulder and waist muscles at the same time.

When the posture is correct, the waist is only one palm (thickness) away from the wall [Figure 11 - 18 (A) and (B)]. If the waist - wall distance is larger than one palm, it indicates that the standing posture is not correct [Figure 11 - 18 (C)].

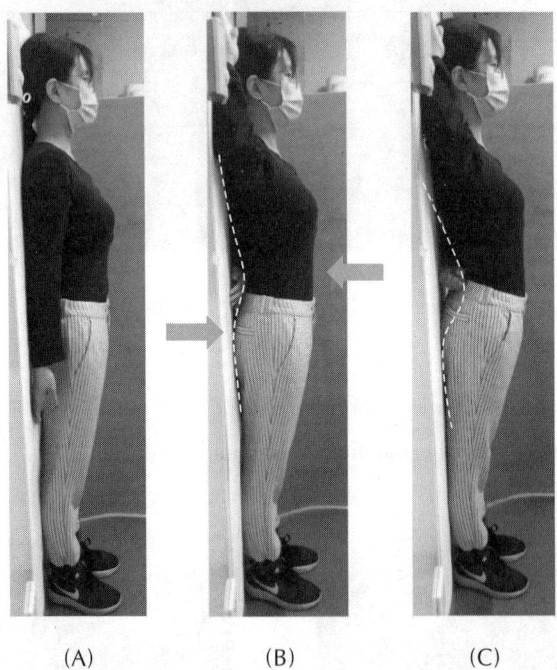

(A) (B) (C)

Figure 11 - 18 Example of standing posture training (A) with comparison between the right gesture (B) and the wrong gesture (C).

Tips

Muscle functional trainings always go with malocclusion treatment.

If there is an existed malocclusion, muscle training alone wouldn't be that effective.

Process assessment for student's practice

The instructor will grade the students' practice according to:

- Class sign in.
- Peer-assessment by other groups.

References

[1] McNamara JA. Influences of respiratory pattern on craniofacial growth [J]. Angle Orthod, 1981, 51 (4): 269-300.

[2] Cheng MC, Enlow DH, Papsidero M, et al. Developmental effects of impaired breathing in the face of the growing child [J]. Angle Orthod, 1988, 58 (4): 309-320.

[3] Jefferson Y. Mouth breathing: adverse effects on facial growth, health, academics, and behavior [J]. Gen Dent, 2010, 58 (1): 18-80.

[4] Proffit WR, Fields HW, Larson BE, et al. Contemporary Orthodontics [M]. 6th ed. St. louis: Mosby Elsevier, 2018.

[5] Kondo E. Muscle Wins!: Treatment in orthodontics [M]. Tokyo: Ishiyaku Publishers, 2007.

[6] Chen YX. Orthodontics foundation, technology and clincal [M]. Beijing: Beijing People's Medical Publishing House, 2012.

[7] McKeown P, Mew J. Cranio-facial changes and mouth breathing [J]. Irish Dental Journal, 2011, 57 (3): 12-18, 17.

CHAPTER 12
APPLICATION OF LASER TECHNIQUES IN PEDIATRIC DENTAL CLINIC

Introduction to laser and its application in pediatric dental clinic

Pediatric dentists try to create a pleasant memory of dental visit for children by using novel, minimally invasive technologies to help children establish life-long positive dental habits. Having a less painful dental experience through the use of a modern technology like laser would be an efficient preventive and therapeutic strategy.

The term laser is an acronym for Light Amplification by Stimulated Emission of Radiation. Laser technology has been introduced into dental field in order to address the therapeutic needs of patients more comfortably and more efficiently. Lasers are classified by the active medium that is used to create the laser energy (Figure 12 - 1). Wavelengths in the range of 193 - 10600 nm are applicable in medicine and dentistry. The wavelength of laser determines its clinical application and type of laser device. The most commonly used lasers in dentistry include neodymium-doped yttrium aluminum garnet (Nd: YAG), carbon dioxide laser (CO_2), erbium-doped yttrium aluminum garnet (Er: YAG), neodymium-doped yttrium aluminum perovskite (Nd: YAP), gallium arsenide (GaAs) (Diode), erbium, chromium-doped yttrium scandium gallium garnet (Er-Cr: YSGG) and argon lasers.

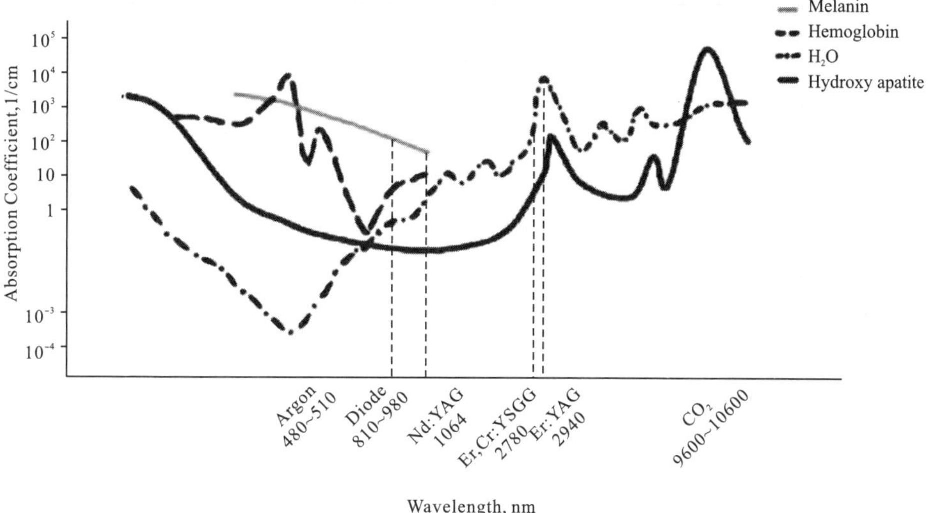

Figure 12 –1 Laser wavelengths and their active medium.

When laser light is absorbed by target tissue, the energy is turned into heat that cuts tissue. The primary action of a laser is absorption in chromophores which is attracted to, i. e. melanin, hemoglobin, water, hydroxy apatite. The photothermal reaction of absorption produces a temperature rise in the target until it expands/vaporizes, and incision/excision occurs.

Clinical applications of lasers in pediatric dental clinic include soft and hard tissue surgery, cavity preparation in the enamel and dentin, detection of dental caries, cleaning the root canal system, etching, caries prevention by changing the crystalline structure of enamel, tooth whitening and periodontal therapy.

Laser must be used with great caution. Adherence to infection control protocol is imperative. Also, reflected or scattered laser beams may be hazardous to unprotected skin and eyes. Wavelength-specific safety goggles must be provided and consistently worn at all times by the dental team, patient, and other observers in attendance during laser use. Local laser safety regulations should be referred by practitioners.

In this particular chapter, we are going to focus on Er: YAG laser and its application in frenum revisions. Laser provides an opportunity for safe correction of an aberrant frenum by removing the fibers causing the problem in a quick office visit, without the need of an operating room or general anesthesia, with less pain than that from a local anesthetic injection, with no need for suturing. A follow-up appointment is scheduled for 5 –7 days later.

The clinical indications for frenum revision in infant, child, and adolescent patients

1. An inability to latch onto mothers' nipples and nurse in newborns.
2. Speech pathology in children.

3. Orthodontic problems in pre-adolescent and adolescent patients.

The objective of lab practice

1. To master the clinical indications for frenum revision in pediatric dental clinic.
2. To master the key points of safe laser use.
3. To be familiar with the procedures of frenum revisions by laser.
4. To know the basic working mechanism of laser.

Materials and instruments

1. Chicken leg with skin [Figure 12 - 2 (A)].
2. Er: YAG laser device [Figure 12 - 2 (B)].
3. Laser handpiece [Figure 12 - 2 (C)].
4. Laser tip [Figure 12 - 2 (C)].
5. Tetracaine hydrochloride gel.
6. Safety goggles [Figure 12 - 2 (D)].
7. Cotton rolls.
8. Iodophor.

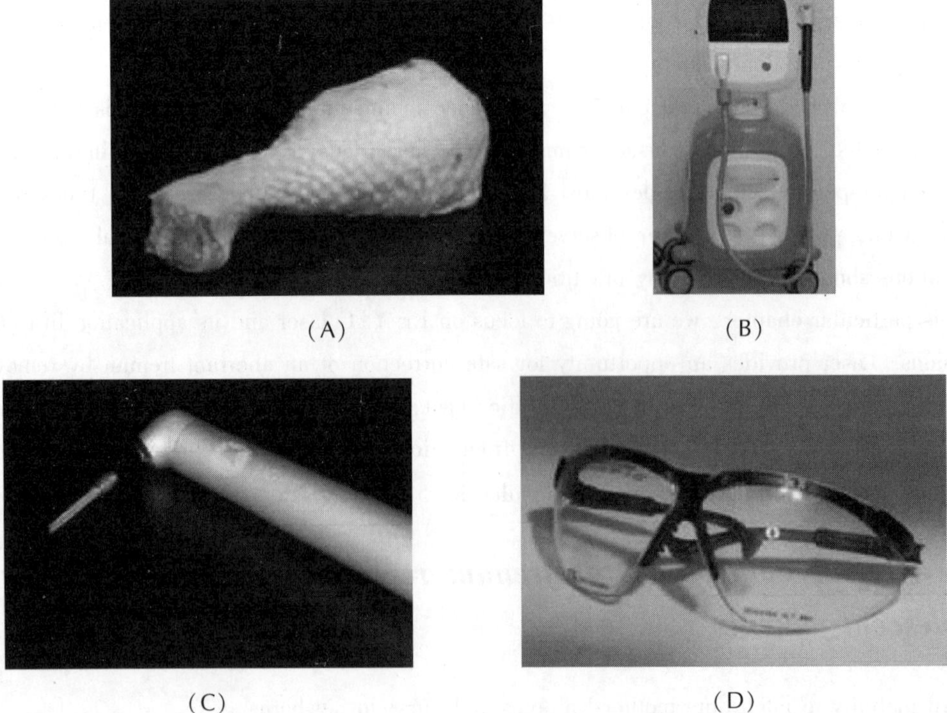

(A) (B) (C) (D)

Figure 12 - 2 Materials and instruments.

Practice steps

1. Set up laser device, handpiece and tip.
2. Set laser parameter at 50 – 150 mJ and 18 – 25 Hz with high water spray [Figure 12 – 3 (A)].
3. Wear safety goggles.
4. Disinfect the operative area with iodophor.
5. Perform topical anesthesia by applying tetracaine hydrochloride gel onto the operative area.
6. When cutting soft tissue using laser, the tip can be either in contact with the tissue, which is similar to using a scalpel, or out of contact with the target, which will cut more slowly at higher powers. Cotton rolls can be used to protect or isolate the operative area [Figure 12 – 3 (B) to (E)].
7. After cutting the extra fibers in the frenum, check the wound. Suturing and hemostasis are usually not needed.

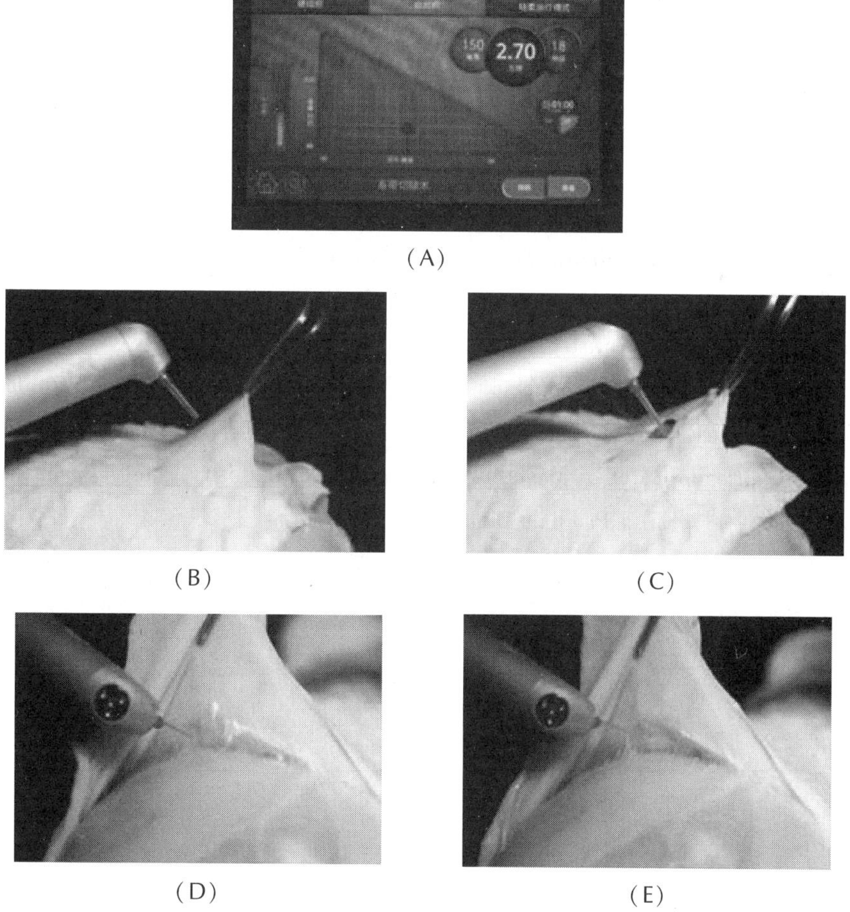

Figure 12 – 3 Laser system set up and practice of soft tissue excision.

Tips

1. When operating with laser, angulation of the beam is critical not only to protect the underlying tissue, but also to keep the tip from being damaged by reflected energy.
2. In clinic, it is important for parents to separate the wound area twice daily by either pulling up the upper lip or pulling down the lower lip to prevent tissue reattachment.
3. In clinic, the follow-up appointment should be scheduled in 5 – 7 days to check the wound healing.

Process assessment for students' practice

The instructor will grade the students' practice according to:

- Proper laser setup and selection of tips.
- Must wear safety goggles.
- Proper setup of laser power and water spray.
- Proper angulation of light beam with target tissue.
- Precise cutting spot and depth.

References

[1] American Academy of Pediatric Dentistry. Policy on the use of lasers for pediatric dental patients [M]. The Reference Manual of Pediatric Dentistry, Chicago: American Academy of Pediatric Dentistry, 2020.

[2] Nazemisalman B, Farsadeghi M, Sokhansanj M. Types of lasers and their applications in pediatric dentistry [J]. J Lasers Med Sci, 2015, 6 (3): 96 – 101.

[3] Olivi G, Caprioglio C, Olivi M, et al. Paediatric laser dentistry. Part 4: Soft tissue laser applications [J]. Eur J Paediatr Dent, 2017, 18 (4): 332 – 334.